CELL BIOLOGY RESEARCH PROGRESS

NEUTROPHILS IN BIOLOGICAL AGE AND LONGEVITY

CELL BIOLOGY RESEARCH PROGRESS

Additional books in this series can be found on Nova's website
under the Series tab.

Additional E-books in this series can be found on Nova's website
under the E-books tab.

CELL BIOLOGY RESEARCH PROGRESS

NEUTROPHILS IN BIOLOGICAL AGE AND LONGEVITY

PATRICIA ALONSO-FERNÁNDEZ,
IANIRE MATÉ
AND
MÓNICA DE LA FUENTE

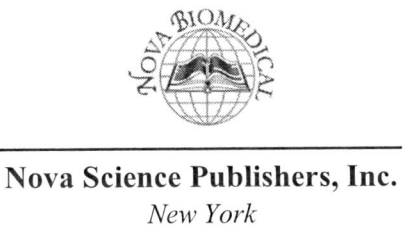

Nova Science Publishers, Inc.
New York

Copyright ©2011 by Nova Science Publishers, Inc.

All rights reserved. No part of this book may be reproduced, stored in a retrieval system or transmitted in any form or by any means: electronic, electrostatic, magnetic, tape, mechanical photocopying, recording or otherwise without the written permission of the Publisher.

For permission to use material from this book please contact us:
Telephone 631-231-7269; Fax 631-231-8175
Web Site: http://www.novapublishers.com

NOTICE TO THE READER

The Publisher has taken reasonable care in the preparation of this book, but makes no expressed or implied warranty of any kind and assumes no responsibility for any errors or omissions. No liability is assumed for incidental or consequential damages in connection with or arising out of information contained in this book. The Publisher shall not be liable for any special, consequential, or exemplary damages resulting, in whole or in part, from the readers' use of, or reliance upon, this material.

Independent verification should be sought for any data, advice or recommendations contained in this book. In addition, no responsibility is assumed by the publisher for any injury and/or damage to persons or property arising from any methods, products, instructions, ideas or otherwise contained in this publication.

This publication is designed to provide accurate and authoritative information with regard to the subject matter covered herein. It is sold with the clear understanding that the Publisher is not engaged in rendering legal or any other professional services. If legal or any other expert assistance is required, the services of a competent person should be sought. FROM A DECLARATION OF PARTICIPANTS JOINTLY ADOPTED BY A COMMITTEE OF THE AMERICAN BAR ASSOCIATION AND A COMMITTEE OF PUBLISHERS.

Library of Congress Cataloging-in-Publication Data

Alonso-Fernandez, Patricia.
  Neutrophils in biological age and longevity / Patricia Alonso-Fernandez,
Ianire Mati, and Msnica de la Fuente.
       p. ; cm.
  Includes bibliographical references and index.
  ISBN 978-1-61728-281-2 (softcover)
  1. Neutrophils. 2. Aging--Immunological aspects. 3. Immune
system--Aging. 4. Aging--Molecular aspects. I. Mati, Ianire. II. Fuente,
Msnica de la. III. Title.
  [DNLM: 1. Neutrophils--immunology. 2. Neutrophils--physiology. 3.
Aging--immunology. 4. Aging--physiology. 5. Longevity--immunology. 6.
Longevity--physiology. WH 200 A454n 2010]
  QR185.8.N47A46 2010
  616.07'9--dc22
                               2010023879

Published by Nova Science Publishers, Inc. ✦ *New York*

Contents

Preface		vii
Chapter 1	Introduction	1
Chapter 2	The Aging Process, Longevity and Biological Age	5
Chapter 3	Theories of Aging. The Integrated Theory of Aging	9
Chapter 4	The Immune System as a Homeostatic System. The Psycho-Neuro-Endocrine-Immune Communication and its Alteration with Aging	13
Chapter 5	Immunosenescence and Age-Related Changes in the Innate Immunity	17
Chapter 6	Functions of Neutrophils and Age-Related Changes	21
Chapter 7	The Immune System, a Marker of Biological Age and Predictor of Longevity	27
Chapter 8	The Role of Oxidative Stress and Inflammatory Stress in Immunosenescence	31
Chapter 9	The Role of the Phagocytic Cells in Oxi-Inflamm-Aging	37
Chapter 10	Influential Factors over the Functional and Redox Parameters in Neutrophils	41
Chapter 11	Neutrophils and their Roles in Disease	47

Chapter 12	Strategies to Revitalize the Neutrophil Functions in Aging	**49**
Chapter 13	Conclusion	**57**
References		**59**
Index		**79**

Preface

Aging is a heterogeneous process in which a progressive and general decrease of the organism's functions leads to a lower ability to adaptively react to changes and preserve homeostasis. Consequently, with aging, there is an increase in vulnerability to age-associated pathologies or, simply, an impairment of functions that leads to death. There are different rates of age-related physiological changes, and the "biological age" determines the level of aging experienced by each individual and, therefore, his/her life expectancy. The age-related impairment of the physiological systems includes the homeostatic systems, such as the immune system, and a fact denominated immunosenescence, which has its basis in the oxidative and imflammatory stress situation. This immunosenescence increases susceptibility to infections, cancer, and autoimmune diseases in old animals, including humans. Moreover, the immune system seems to be involved in the chronic oxy-inflamm-aging. It has been proposed that the functional capacity of the immune cells is a marker of health and longevity. Phagocytic cells, especially neutrophils, act in the early phase of defense against infecting microorganisms. In order to carry out their function, neutrophils need to produce oxidant and pro-inflammatory compounds. It is known that all cells, including immune cells, require adequate levels of antioxidant defenses to prevent damage to biomolecules caused by the excess of oxidation. Thus, to maintain appropriate levels of antioxidants, such as glutathione, and the activity of antioxidant enzymes, such as catalase, it is very important to avoid oxidation and the resulting inactivation of lipid and DNA in immune cells. We have analyzed several function and redox parameters in peripheral blood neutrophils from healthy men and women of different ages, as well as in centenarians, and compared them with healthy younger groups. We have also analyzed if gender differences, seasonal changes, and circadian changes can influence those parameters. We have proposed that the age-related oxidative stress in the immune cells, especially in phagocytic cells, could be responsible for the impairment of the immune functions and the increase in chronic oxidative stress of the organisms. Moreover, these immune cells could modulate the rate of aging. Therefore, the functional parameters studied in neutrophils may be useful markers of "biological age" and predictors of longevity.

Chapter 1

Introduction

Aging is a heterogeneous process characterized by a time-related decline in physiological functions. It affects many components of the organism and supposes a reduction of the homeostasis, the adaptive capacity and a loss of response capacity to changes. The consequence is an increase in vulnerability and the development of age-associated pathologies or just the impairment of functions that leads to death. Aging supposes a continuous adaptation of the body, including the immune system, to impairments that occur over time, with some mechanisms deteriorating and others being maintained or stimulated[1].

There are different rates of age-related physiological changes. Tissues age at different rates, and individuals with the same chronological age have different rates of aging. For this reason, the "Biological Age" is a better indicator of the rate of aging in each subject than the chronological age[1]. It has been proposed that biological age determines the level of aging experienced by each individual and may serve as an indicator of an individual's general health status, remaining healthy life span and active life expectancy[2].

Immunosenescence, the progressive age-related impairment of immune function[3, 4], renders the aged more susceptible to infectious diseases, resulting in increased morbidity and mortality. Elderly people constitute the most rapidly increasing segment in Europe and the U.S. Older adults exhibit a heightened incidence of infectious disease, a major cause of death in the elderly (especially influenza, pneumonia and urinary tract infections)[5-8]. With the the increased rates of infectious disease, autoimmune disorders, inappropriate inflammatory conditions and cancer, they consequently present the highest health care costs per capita[8, 9]. Thus, a thorough understanding of the mechanisms responsible for age-related declines in immune function and the need to identify and implement strategies to counteract immunosenescence is a pressing issue, with physicians and researchers actively investigating possible compensatory therapies.

Immunosenescence is not an inevitable decline of all immune functions. It is the result of a continuous remodeling process where several functions are decreased, while others remain unchanged, or are even increased[10]. While most studies have focused on age-related declines in immune function, it is more accurate to think of immunosenescence as a state of dysregulation, because leucocytes respond heterogeneously to aging.

Immunity is classically conceptualized as two distinct but interacting systems: innate and adaptive, and immunosenescence affects both[11-14]. Innate immunity could be named the basal or first immune response. It includes both cellular and chemical systems, and it is responsible for the rapid and automatically activated response to the threat. If innate immunity is not adequate and a more specialized defense is required, adaptive immunity is launched. Adaptive immunity utilizes innate immunity in its attack, but also develops additional responses specific to the particular invader. There are several important differences between innate and adaptive immunity. While innate immunity may act within seconds of detecting a threat, the construction of a specialized adaptive immune response generally requires 2–5 days. Repeated exposure to a given pathogen will enhance the adaptive immune response, but not the innate, because only adaptive immunity has immunological memory.

In the present chapter we are going to discuss how the study of functional, redox and inflammatory state parameters of phagocytic cells from high longevity subjects (human centenarians and extremely long-living mice), as well as from mice with premature aging, show the role of these immune cells as markers of biological age and predictors of longevity. Moreover, the phagocytic cells could show the effects of environmental and lifestyle factors in the maintenance of homeostasis in each subject in the context of the communication among the physiological regulatory systems, namely the immune, nervous and endocrine systems. In addition, these could be the cells most directly involved in the rate of aging, and consequently, in the longevity of each individual (Figure 1).

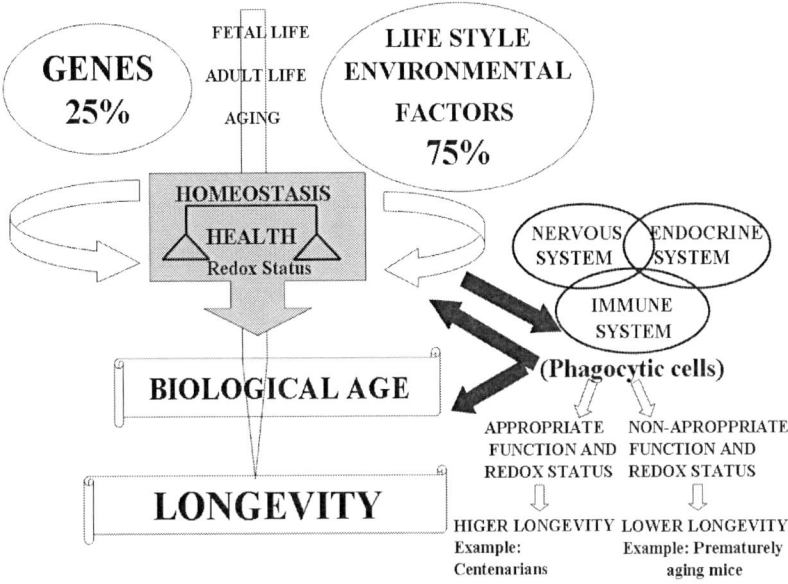

Figure 1. The basis of functional longevity is health maintenance, and this depends on the preservation of homeostasis (the balance at all physiological levels). This health preservation depends, approximately, on a proportion in which 25% is genetic factors, but 75% depends upon the style of life and environmental factors. These epigenetic mechanisms act on genes during fetal life and throughout the life of the subject. With aging there is impairment of the regulatory systems, namely the nervous, the endocrine and the immune systems, as well as of the neuro-endocrine-immune communication. These age-related alterations lead to loss of homeostasis and, therefore, to an increase in morbidity and mortality. This loss of homeostasis is established at a different rate in each subject, determining its biological age. Since the functional and redox states of the immune system, and concretely of the phagocytic cells, are good markers of health, biological age and predictors of longevity, we propose their study in order to determine each particular rate of aging and its response to changes in the style of life and environmental factors. Moreover, there is a relation between the oxidative state of leukocytes, their function and individual longevity. Thus, high levels of oxidative stress in the phagocytic cells result in an impaired function and a lower longevity of the subjects that have these cells. This has been found in peritoneal macrophages from prematurely aging mice (PAM), a model based on the higher anxiety levels of these animals. On the contrary, low oxidative stress in phagocytic cells is accompanied by better function of these cells and by high longevity of the subjects, as we have observed in macrophages of long-living mice and in neutrophils of centenarians.

Chapter 2

The Aging Process, Longevity and Biological Age

Definition of Aging

Aging may be defined as a progressive and general decrease of the organism's functions that leads to a lower ability to adaptively react to changes and preserve homeostasis. This accumulation of adverse changes, as a consequence of the passage of time, increases the risk of disease and finally results in death. Thus, although aging should not be considered a disease, it strongly increases the chances of suffering many degenerative diseases. As Strehler[15] pointed out, there are four rules that define aging. It is universal (practically all animal species, including the metazoans, showing sexual reproduction suffer aging); progressive (the rate of aging is similar at different ages after the adult state); intrinsic (the causes must be endogenous since even if animals are exposed to optimal environmental conditions throughout life, they still experience the aging process at the rate characteristic for their species); and deleterious (aging is obviously detrimental to the individual since it leads to their death). However, at the species level, the detrimental character of aging could be argued since it is counteracted by a continuous replacement of the members of the population.

Longevity

The aging process is finished at the end of the maximum lifespan or maximum longevity, the maximum time that a subject belonging to a determined species can live. In human beings, for instance, it is about 122 years, whereas in mouse and rat strains it is only 3 and 4 years respectively. It is very important to distinguish the maximum lifespan from the mean longevity or mean lifespan, which can be defined as the mean of time that the members of a population who have been born on the same date will live. The maximum longevity is fixed in each species, but the mean lifespan of individual organisms, even when they are of the same genotype and are raised in a common environment protected from extrinsic hazards, shows marked variability[16]. Although it is presently impossible to increase the maximum longevity, the mean lifespan can be increased by environmental factors that allow organisms to maintain good health and approach the maximum lifespan in good condition. Thus, presently, human aging is a problem in terms of the cost of health care in developed countries because the mean longevity is very high, about 75-83 years. Since we start the aging process at about 18 years old, we spend most time of our life aging. Because of this, it is very important to know which factors of lifestyle can increase this longevity and how they can do it. A higher mean longevity is achieved by preservation of good health and this depends on a proportion in which approximately 25% is genetic and 75% is the style of life and environmental factors[17] (Figure 1).

Biological Age

The aging process is very heterogeneous. Thus, there are different rates of physiological changes in the different systems of the organism and in the different members of a population of the same chronological age. This justifies the introduction of the concept of "biological age," which is very useful in assessing the level of aging experienced by each individual and, therefore, his life expectancy. Since chronological age fails to provide an accurate indicator of the aging process[18] and aging is associated with a great number of changes in all levels of biological organization, there is a need to select parameters that are useful as biomarkers of aging. The most complete investigation on biological age was performed by Borkan and Norris[1], on over one thousand men, in the longitudinal study on human aging of the

Gerontological Center of Baltimore. The retrospective analysis of this study showed that the subjects presenting certain parameters aged more than those found in the majority of the subjects of the same chronological age and had a shorter life expectancy. These biomarkers include those related to respiratory function, systolic arterial tension and reaction times determined by psychometric tests. Although the concept of biological aging has been investigated since the 1970s, most studies mainly selected a profile of physical parameters, including some physiological and biochemical parameters, and in spite of recent attempts to extend the kinds of parameters of biological age[19], the proposals are still incomplete. Thus, most research on biological age did not include immune parameters. Since the immune function is a marker of health and longevity[20] and a positive relation has been shown between a good function of several immune cells and longevity[21-26], several immune parameters are considered essential and very representative of the biological age of a subject, and, thus, they can be considered appropriate biomarkers of biological age (as reviewed in more detail below).

Chapter 3

Theories of Aging. The Integrated Theory of Aging

How does aging happen?, Where does aging start? Why does aging occur? The answers to these key questions in gerontology have stimulated such an amount of speculation to justify the critical comment that there are as many theories of aging as there are gerontologists. Thus, as consequence of the great complexity of changes associated with senescence, more than 300 theories have been proposed to explain the process of aging[27]. Currently most of these theories have been abandoned since they do not agree with the data from research on humans and research animals, whereas other theories find acceptance and are supported by research.

Although the theories of senescence proposed are too numerous to enumerate and several kinds of classifications of these theories have been published[28, 29], we feel that most of these theories can be joined in three groups. "Genetic program theories" propose that aging is the result of a purposeful program driven by the genes. In another group are the "epigenetic theories," which indicate that aging is the result of events that are not guided by a genetic program but are stochastic or random events. The third group corresponds to the "evolutionary theories of aging," which do not try to explain the mechanism of aging, but instead attempt to explain why the aging process occurs and the reasons for the different rates of aging in the different species. In the first group we can include those theories proposing the existence of specific genes of longevity, theories of existence of biological clocks for aging[30], or the shortening telomere theory (telomere attrition occurs with each round of cell division)[27, 31]. Many of these theories have been considered as possible explanations of cell differentiation processes or replicative cellular senescence, but not the basis of organism aging. In the epigenetic group, it is possible to include several groups of theories: a) molecular structural stabilization and cross-linkage theories; b) metabolic theories (aging can be considered "a side effect" of aerobic metabolism: "*wear- and- tear*" or disorganization, rate-of-living, oxidation, damage by free radical, mitochondrial injury)[27, 29, 32]; and c) physiological theories of aging, in which the neuroendocrine and the immunological theories are included[27]. In the group of evolutionary theories we can mention theories such as the risk of depredation, duration of development, rate of reproduction, and others[27, 28]. The first evolutionary theory of senescence, which was suggested by Weissman[27, 33], considered aging necessary for the disposal of the mortal soma in order to prevent organisms from competing with their progeny for food and space.

Nowadays, despite the claims of some researchers, there is no direct evidence that only the genes drive age changes. Even researchers following genetic theories in the past are now defenders of the idea that the aging process, which appears after reproductive maturation, is driven by random events and not gene-programmed[34]. In conclusion, most theories of aging explain events that are consequences of the aging process but not their cause. Several of the epigenetic theories and evolutionary theories are useful in trying to solve the puzzle of aging, and we will use them further to elaborate an integrated theory of aging.

The Integrated Theory of Aging

Since the aging process is very complex, a theory based on only one mechanism cannot offer a satisfactory explanation of all its aspects. This justifies the proposal of a theory that integrates early concepts that offer partial explanations of the mechanism of aging with other, more recent concepts[32, 33, 35-39] (Table 2). Thus, an integrated theory has been recently proposed which attempts to reply to the three important questions of biogerontology: the how, where and why of aging[40]. Regarding the question of how, the aging process is linked to the oxidation produced by the oxidative stress, which is the cause of many age-related changes that affect a large number of parameters, including morphology, physiology and behaviour at all levels of organization (molecular, cellular, tissues, organs and systems). A reasonable answer to the question of where aging starts is in the mitochondria from fixed differentiated cells, as first proposed by Miquel et al.[35]. As for the question of why does aging happens, the answer seems to be found in several evolutionary theories such as the concept of Williams[39] that aging is a consequence of characteristics selected by evolution as an advantage for the young subjects of the species, allowing them to reach the reproductive age in the best condition and thus preserve these species, but which are a disadvantage for older subjects. Thus, the selection acts before the adult age, and the maintenance of the species is more relevant biologically than the longevity of the individual. Moreover, it is evident that what allows for better functioning in the age of reproduction, namely oxygen utilization for cell energy production, is the main cause of functional impairment afterwards. Thus aging would be an unprogrammed effect of high levels of oxidative stress in the differentiated cells, quite irrelevant from the viewpoint of species survival through sexual reproduction.

Chapter 4

The Immune System as a Homeostatic System. The Psycho-Neuro-Endocrine-Immune Communication and its Alteration with Aging

The immune system is one of the regulatory systems of the organism, contributing to homeostasis by recognizing and eliminating foreign and altered self-antigens, thus maintaining the appropriate cell types and molecules that constitute the tissues and organs. The immune system is a remarkably versatile defense system that has evolved to protect animals from infectious agents (e.g. bacteria, viruses, fungi, parasites, etc) and malignant cells. This activity is carried out, from the birth of the individual, via different components such as epithelial barriers, immune cells and immune molecules, which act together in a dynamic and complexity network. The immune system is constantly active in order to discriminate "non-self" from "self" and, thus, destroy the non-self. Moreover, this system, with its cells and mediators, contributes to the maintenance of the correct functions of the body[41, 42]. Thus, the appropriate functioning of the immune system has been considered the best marker of health and longevity[20, 42, 43].

Two types of immunity protect the body: innate (or natural, non-specific) and adaptive (or acquired, specific). Innate immunity consists of cells such as dendritic cells (DCs), macrophages, natural killer cells (NKs), and neutrophils, as well as molecular systems such as complement and cytokines. This innate immunity is already present at birth and provides the first barrier against invaders. If pathogens pass the epithelial and mucosal barriers, the above mentioned cells come into play rapidly to eliminate them, and, hence, contain the infections. In addition, NK cells are also implicated in the control of infections and resistance to tumors, destroying infected cells and tumor cells through cytotoxic granule release, similar to the activity of T cells (though in a nonspecific way). Macrophages are other leucocytes belonging to the innate immune system that serve four important roles. They present antigens (molecules of pathogens or tumor cells recognized as foreign) to memory (but not naïve) cells, produce both cytokines and reactive nitrogen and oxygen species, and clean up cellular debris. The basic signaling receptors of the innate immune cells in the recognition of pathogens are the Toll-like receptors (TLR), which detect a broad range of molecular patterns that are commonly found on pathogens, called pathogen-associated molecular patterns (PAMPs).

With regard to the adaptive immunity, this is a more sophisticated immunity. It is performed by lymphocytes, which act when the innate defense cannot clear the infection in a short time. This immunity involves the specific recognition of antigens. Communication within the adaptive immunity and between innate and acquired systems requires direct cell-to-cell interactions, as well as the production of chemical messengers such as cytokines. Thus, DCs reside in the lymphoid tissues and serve as storehouses and presenters of antigens to activate B and T cells; thus, DCs are important in initiating adaptive immune responses. Macrophages, like DCs, also link innate and adaptive immunity.

The Psycho-Neuro-Immune Communication

It is recognized that the nervous and the immune systems are linked and involved in a bidirectional communication. The concept of nervous system modulation of immunological and inflammatory responses is supported by the identification of neurotransmitter receptors on leukocytes and by the increasing number of findings showing that the nervous mediators can regulate immune functions. In addition, cytokines produced by the immune cells act on the nervous system, whose cells are receptors for the immune mediators. Thus, there is a "neuroendocrine-immune" system that allows for the preservation of homeostasis and therefore of health[44-46] (Figure 1). It was suggested that the immune system represents a system of information reception of non-cognition related stimuli that appears in the organism (infections, tumor cells or other types of foreign cells) and response to those stimuli. It is accompanied by the transfer of that information (through cytokines produced by immune cells) to the neuroendocrine system. On the other hand, the neuroendocrine system is a receptor of cognitive stimuli (light, sound, stress situations, etc.) to which it responds. Its mediators (neurotransmitters and hormones) reach the immune system to inform it about the situation[47]. The scientific confirmation of this communication has allowed understanding of, on the basis of the experimental data, a number of facts of everyday life. Thus, it is well known that situations of depression, emotional stress, or anxiety are accompanied by a greater vulnerability to conditions, ranging from infectious processes to cancer or autoimmune diseases, which agrees with the concept that the immune system is impaired and it results in worse health and a shorter life span[48, 49]. By contrast, pleasant emotions and an "optimistic outlook" on life help us to overcome immune system-related diseases and enjoy better overall health[50]. Conversely, it has been shown that immune system changes, such as those found in infectious processes, alter nervous system functions, which can even lead to psychotic disorders and neural diseases[51].

With age all regulatory systems involved in homeostasis (for example, the nervous, the endocrine and the immune system), as well as the communication between them, show an impairment[41, 42, 52]. This important observation justified the proposal of another theory of aging, according to changes in this communication between the immune system and the nervous system with age (and concomitant loss of homeostasis and resistance to stress), that is the probable cause of physiological senescence[53]. Recent studies of our group support this hypothesis, as well as the idea that the immunosenescence could affect functions of other regulatory systems through an increased oxidative and inflammatory stress, resulting in the age-related homeostasis alteration and increase in morbidity and mortality[41, 42].

Chapter 5

Immunosenescence and Age-Related Changes in the Innate Immunity

Immunosenescence

As mentioned above, aging is accompanied by a decline of the physiological systems, including the immune functions. In fact, it is well known that time action produces a decrease in the resistance to infections and an increase in autoimmune processes and cancer, which indicates the presence of a less competent immune system. In fact, the increased death rate found in aged populations is due in great proportion to infectious processes[54]. Thus, there is an impairment of the immune system with age, which exerts a great influence on the increasing morbidity and mortality observed in aging human subjects[20]. Nowadays it is accepted, although there are conflicting observations on this subject, that almost every component of the immune system undergoes striking age-associated re-structuring, leading to changes that may include enhanced, as well as diminished, functions involving each component of the immune system, as well as their interactions[41-43, 55-59]. This fact is denominated immunosenescence.

Immunosenescence results in a pronounced decrease in T-cell functions, especially in the T-cell helper, which affects humoral immunity and causes an impaired B-cell function[57, 58, 60]. However, not all immune cell types or all functions of an immune cell show a significant decrease. In fact, several cell types and functions are activated with age, whereas other types and functions do not show significant age-related changes. Thus, a cell type which has been relatively neglected in studies of age and immunity is the Treg subset. With age these cells maintain their functional capacity but increase in number, and this could explain the greater suppressive activity in the elderly[61, 62].

Age-related alterations in innate immunity cells have been studied less than lymphocytes. Although the evidence accumulated over the last decade supports the profound impact of aging on innate immunity, the results obtained on the age-related changes of the functions of cells from innate immunity are often contradictory[42, 55, 56, 63-67].

In addition, since the innate and adaptive immune systems cooperate to ensure an optimal immune response, we have to consider that any decline in innate immunity will impact the function of the adaptive immune system and vice versa[42, 63, 67, 68]. Thus, at the level of a key component of T cell immunity, as is the antigen presentation, the age-related changes in the antigen presenting cells, such as macrophages and dendritic cells, could play a relevant role in the alterations of the initiation and outcome of T cell immune response[63]. Moreover, the dendritic cells have been implicated in the age-related change to a predominant Th2 response instead of the predominant Th1 of the adult[69]. In fact, this change from predominant Th1-type to predominant Th2-type responses to antigens with an accompanying shift in cytokine profiles has been proposed as a mechanism for age-related immune dysfunction[60].

Although several of the age-related changes observed in the immune response have been attributed to the modifications of immune cell subpopulations with aging[60, 70], the age-related quantitative variations in a type of immune cell is not necessarily related to its function. For example, NK cells increase in number with age, but decrease their cytotoxic capacity[60, 63, 70]. However, the presence of a higher ratio of memory lymphocytes with respect to naive cells could explain the decrease of several immune functions[60, 69]. Despite the fast increasing amount of data on immunosenescence[55-72], the puzzle of all the changes in the different aspects of the immune function with age has not been solved yet, and the specific role played by the immune system in aging of organisms is not wholly understood.

Age-Related Changes in the Innate Immunity

Several aspects of the innate immune response are affected by normal human aging, resulting in a reduced ability to provide the immediate response to bacterial and viral pathogens and also to integrate with the adaptive immune response. The mechanisms underlying these changes are now beginning to be characterized and include alterations in the activity of a variety of innate immune cell receptors and their downstream signaling pathways, as well as changes in the numbers and functional capacity of certain cells within the circulation. Thus, this loss of innate cell function has consequences for immunity and longevity[73-76].

In general, the NK cells, one of the cellular mediators of innate defense more extensively studied in the elderly, show a decreased cytotoxicity and cytokine production[63, 66]. Circulating numbers of NK cells increase with age and total NK cell pool activity appears to be maintained with aging; however, the per se killing capacities and IFN-gamma producing capacities of these cells appears to be impaired, perhaps due to an age-associated shift towards a "mature phenotype"[77-79].

The effects of aging on DC responses have not been studied extensively; however, some of the published data suggest that aging tends to be associated with a decrease of several specific functions of certain types of DCs[80].

The phagocytic cells such as macrophages and monocytes show a significant decrease in several of their functions[25, 26, 42, 63-67, 72, 81]. Thus, although phagocytes were thought to play a less critical role in the immune dysfunction that occurs over time, recent studies point to the general decline in the functional activities of these cells as one major reason for the susceptibility and vulnerability to bacterial and viral infections among aged subjects, which stand out as the most common causes of illness and death in aging[42, 63-67]. Immunosenescence is associated with a general decline in macrophage function [56], possibly due to impaired ability of macrophages to respond to activation or due to a decline in activation signals from other cells. The antigen-presenting capacities of peripheral blood monocytes from older humans appear to be compromised due to alterations in MHC class II gene expression[82], and the activities of infection-response proteins, such as heat shock proteins, may also be altered[83]. Aging has been associated with alterations in the pro-inflammatory/anti-inflammatory cytokine release balance. Monocytes and macrophages, as well as other cell types, can produce pro-inflammatory cytokines such as IL-1, IL-6, and tumor necrosis factor-α (TNF-α. Although results from numerous studies suggest that serum levels of pro-inflammatory cytokines are increased with advancing age, it is less clear whether LPS-stimulated or pathogen-induced production of IL-1, IL-6 or TNF-α by monocytes/macrophages (or both) are altered with age. Presently it is accepted that adherence capacity, expression of Toll-like receptors such as TLR2 or TLR4, or production of pro-inflammatory cytokines, are increased with aging[41, 42, 65, 66].

Chapter 6

Functions oF Neutrophils and Age-Related Changes

Functions of Neutrophils

Neutrophils are the most prevalent white blood cell in human blood. As phagocytic granulocytes, they play an important role in consuming (through phagocytosis) and/or destroying (through granule release) extracellular pathogens. Thus, these cells act in the early phase of defense against infecting microorganisms. Neutrophils are among the first cells to be recruited at the site of any inflammatory insult and are the first cells to participate in the phagocytic process, which consists of several stages. The first stage involves adherence to the vascular endothelium, before transmigration to the extravascular space along concentration gradients of chemokines (chemotaxis)[84]. Endothelial dysfunction, arising in part through interaction with activated neutrophils, may be critical to the development of sepsis syndromes[85]. When the neutrophils reach the infecting microorganisms, their phagocytosis function begins. This function is the most representative and relevant of these cells. At the focus of infection, apoptosis of the neutrophils (short-lived cells with a half-life of only 8–12 hours in peripheral blood) is delayed by the intervention of factors such as bacterial stimuli [formyl-methionyl-leucyl-phenylalanine (fMLP) and lipopolisacharide (LPS)], complement, and pro-inflammatory cytokines ,such as tumour necrosis factor alfa (TNF-α)[86], and granulocyte macrophage-colony stimulating factor (GM-CSF)[87, 88]. Without this intervention, many neutrophils would die shortly after arrival at the site of inflammation. Locally mediated activation initiates the neutrophil oxidative burst, producing ROS. In this phagocytic process, the destruction of the ingested material frequently involves the production of protease enzymes and other pro-inflammatory mediators, which are also released by degranulation and have bactericidal and fungicidal properties, which are relevant to the inflammatory reaction. ROS and proteases damage cells, extracellular matrix proteins and other macromolecules, whereas cytokine release maintains the influx of inflammatory cells, thereby perpetuating the response. The activated neutrophils produce high volumes of microbicidal and pathogenic ROS. The later induction of apoptosis by ROS may therefore be of fundamental importance to neutrophils' removal from a site of inflammation, representing a potential mechanism of negative feedback in the inflammatory response. Neutrophils die by apoptosis, but if the number of apoptotic neutrophils at the inflamed site exceeds the capacity of macrophages to clear the dead cells, they could progress to secondary necrosis, leading to persistence of inflammation[89]. Following an encounter and subsequent phagocytosis of pathogens, the neutrophil oxidative burst leads to apoptosis not only of the engulfing cell, but also of those in close approximation.

At sites of inflammation, neutrophils encounter an environment in which the usual balance between pro-oxidant and antioxidant molecules may be upset. As it has been seen, the phagocytic process and destruction of the ingested material involves the production of oxygen-free radicals, the first of which is superoxide anion, a precursor of active microbicidal oxidants[90]. Most cells deploy a range of mechanisms for the maintenance of redox balance in the face of excessive pro-oxidant stress. Because of the high levels of pro-oxidant species generated by the local tissues and by neutrophils themselves, these immune cells require adequate levels of antioxidant defenses to prevent damage to biomolecules caused by the excess of free radicals. Moreover, leukocytes are particularly sensitive to oxidative damage because of the high content of polyunsaturated fatty acids in their membranes and the genetic expression required for their defense function[91]. More subtle modulation of redox balance may contribute to the physiological regulation of intracellular signaling, including several of the distal pathways involved in the execution of apoptosis[92]. The neutrophil maintains a number of systems for the regulation of redox balance, including catalase and GSH [93,94]. In neutrophils cultured for more than 24 h these antioxidant substances become depleted, thus promoting a pro-oxidant and, therefore, pro-apoptotic state[95]. Separate investigation with GSH-depleting agents has confirmed that altering the redox environment results in a predisposition to apoptosis[96]. GSH depletion during activation of the respiratory burst has also been demonstrated and would facilitate apoptosis seen following phagocytosis[97]. Fas receptor activation leads to increased GSH efflux and apoptosis in nonneutrophil cell lines[98], whereas increase of intracellular GSH in neutrophils inhibits apoptosis[99]. The relative inability of mature neutrophils to promote *de novo* synthesis of protein may contribute to the rapid decrease of GSH seen with both physiological and pathological levels of oxidative stress. This fall in GSH and subsequent increase in ROS may contribute to the initiation of spontaneous apoptosis[100]. Thus, to maintain appropriate levels of antioxidants, such as glutathione, and adequate levels of the activity of antioxidant enzymes, such as catalase, it is very important to avoid oxidation and the resulting inactivation of lipids and DNA in immune cells.

Neutrophils' Functions and Aging

In order to describe the effect of aging over the different neutrophils' functions, we analyze the most-representative functions of peripheral blood neutrophils in healthy middle-aged adults, and we compare them with those of healthy young adults[101]. In addition we studied those functions in healthy centenarians and compared them with young healthy adults[101]. To avoid confounding factors such as chronic disease, nutrition, and lifestyle that have a profound effect on immunity and thus conceal more-subtle age-related changes, we worked under the SENIEUR EURAGE protocol, which sets strict inclusion criteria for human immunogerontology studies that include clinical information, laboratory data, and immunopharmacological interferences[102].

With aging, neutrophils show greater adherence to endothelium and lower chemotaxis capacity (Figure 2). In several studies carried out, by us and other authors, this greater adhesion of neutrophils from elderly subjects has been shown[41, 66, 68]. This high adherence to endothelium does not allow them to perform their function appropriately. Both alterations (adherence and chemotaxis) have also been observed in other phagocytic cells, such as macrophages, from aging mice[26, 65, 103]. Moreover, peritoneal macrophages from prematurely aging mice (PAM) show greater adherence and lower chemotaxis than nonprematurely aging mice (NPAM) of the same chronological age, and PAM have a shorter life span than NPAM. Some studies have reported an increase in adhesion molecule expression[104] and plasma membrane fluidity associated with aging, related to a decrease in cholesterol content, in peritoneal neutrophils from aged rats. These altered functions[105] were related to greater oxidative stress[41, 106] and are associated with a 40% decrease in superoxide generation in response to the bacterial peptide fMLP[105]. However, the superoxide response to the phorbol ester phorbol myristic acid (PMA), which activates downstream signaling events via direct activation of protein kinase C (PKC), was not affected, suggesting a defect proximal to the receptor. Alterations of membrane fluidity would thus impact on lipid raft formation and integrity with consequences for a range of membrane receptors. Lipid rafts are regions of reduced fluidity within the phospholipid bilayer and are enriched in cholesterol and phospholipids with long, saturated fatty acid side chains. Lipid rafts are important for the regulation of cell signaling because they provide a means to segregate receptors and their proximal signaling components within the membrane, with receptor activity modulated by the inclusion or exclusion of signaling elements in the lipid raft associated signalosome[107]. Although similar studies of the lipid composition of neutrophils from old humans have not been reported, there is evidence that lipid raft function might be compromised in human neutrophils with age. Indeed, the negative regulator of GM-CSF receptor signaling SHP-1 is excluded from lipid rafts within 1 minute of stimulation of young neutrophils with GM-CSF but remains associated with lipid rafts in neutrophils from old donors[108], thus maintaining inhibition of receptor signaling. At the same time, agonist receptors such as TREM-1 and TLR4 show reduced recruitment to lipid rafts in neutrophils of aging donors, compromising their signaling function[89, 109]. Taken together, these data might explain the reduction in downstream signaling events in old neutrophils[89, 110, 111] mediating superoxide generation, chemotaxis and antiapoptotic processes110.

Many of the defects in neutrophil function might arise from changes on the cell membrane and/or to proximal events in receptor signaling. For example, neutrophil priming and activation in response to a range of ligands is decreased with age, including fMLP, GM-CSF, granulocyte-colony stimulating factor (G-CSF) and LPS[87], as is the response to ligation of the neutrophil receptor TREM-1[89]. Overall, these data suggest that changes in membrane fluidity seen with age could provide a general mechanism for many of the dysfunctional signaling pathways seen in neutrophils from the elderly[112].

In regard to chemotactic activity, neutrophils from elderly subjects show lower chemotactic activity[41, 68, 74, 113, 114]. When neutrophils are adherent to endothelium and have very low migration capacity toward the infectious focus, they cannot perform their function appropriately. The efficiency of migration to the infected site could thus be affected as a result of reduced chemotactic ability, and some studies have shown that this is associated with increased morbidity and mortality in aged patients with infections after trauma[74, 115]. For instance, the increased adherence and reduced chemotaxis of neutrophils with age could contribute to the higher risk of infections in elderly people[116]. Also peritoneal macrophages from prematurely aging mice (PAM) show lower chemotaxis than nonprematurely aging mice (NPAM) of the same chronological age, and PAM have a shorter life span than NPAM[117]. The movement of neutrophils toward a site of inflammation is affected by two components of migration, namely chemokinesis (speed of movement) and chemotaxis (directional movement). To date, only a single study has assessed the effect of age on both elements of neutrophil migration, and the data indicate that chemokinesis is intact but chemotaxis is reduced with age[114]. As neutrophils migrate toward a site of infection, their movement through tissues is affected by the release of proteases, such as elastase. Once in the tissue, the age-related decrease in chemotactic ability[74, 114] could result in increased collateral damage to healthy tissues due to reduced directional movement and persistence toward the site of infection, reduced phagocytic function and bactericidal activity (superoxide generation), and inability to extend neutrophil lifespan via inflammatory survival factors. All of these will compromise the efficiency of removal of microbes and thus extend the time to resolve the inflammation. Moreover, an association between low chemotaxis and high lipid peroxide levels with high mortality has been observed[74].

With respect to the ingestion and microbiocidal capacities of neutrophils, both decrease with age[101] (Figure 2). Neutrophils from elderly humans are less phagocytic than those from younger adults[68, 101, 114, 118]. Moreover, a lower ingestion capacity in phagocytic cells would allow greater development of infection, and previous results have shown that a reduced life span accompanies impaired phagocytosis by peritoneal macrophages from PAM[25, 26, 117]. The respiratory burst has been shown to be altered in neutrophils from aged volunteers. Superoxide (O_2-) and hydrogen peroxide (H_2O_2) production in vitro by neutrophils from aged humans is increased[68, 101] when compared to cells from young humans. Superoxide anion production by neutrophils is necessary for the digestion of ingested material, but excessive production of this free radical is often harmful when it is not compensated by antioxidant defenses, because it may induce not only bacterial killing, but also tissue damage if it is present at high levels[119]. Several studies have found higher levels of superoxide anions in macrophages from old mice than from young adult mice[25], as well as in neutrophils from elderly subjects[66, 120]. Moreover, lower levels of reactive oxygen species have been reported in longer-living strains of houseflies and mice[121, 122].

In relation to the molecular mechanisms involved in these age-related alterations in neutrophil function, the alteration in intracellular signaling following receptor ligation helps to explain decreased phagocytosis capacity in neutrophils from the elderly. In fact, some studies have shown that the decreased intracellular Ca2+ after fMLP stimulation may help to explain reduced phagocytic ability[123] and decreased bactericidal activity[114]. Actin polymerization is markedly reduced after stimulation of neutrophils from aged subjects with fMLP or phorbol myristate acetate (PMA) – an activator of protein kinase C (PKC) – relative to younger subjects[124], and this has been associated with impaired O2- production[125]. A reduction in the ability of neutrophils from the elderly to be primed by GMCSF or to activate the respiratory burst has been extensively documented[110]. Triggering receptor expressed on myeloid cell-1 (TREM-1) is a receptor with important roles in diverse neutrophil functions, such as phagocytosis, respiratory burst and degranulation[126], as has been demonstrated in neutrophils obtained from aged humans. Following TREM-1 engagement, neutrophils from aged donors had diminished respiratory burst relative to neutrophils from younger donors[89]. In addition, the phosphorylation of TREM-1 effectors, such as AKT and phospholipase C-c, was also altered with aging[89]. Taken together, these results indicate that age affects the microbiocidal capacity of neutrophils.

Chapter 7

The Immune System, a Marker of Biological Age and Predictor of Longevity

It has been demonstrated that the competence of the immune system is an excellent marker of health[20], and several age-related changes in immune functions have been linked to longevity[21-26, 41, 42]. Thus, parameters such as excess of CD8+ CD27- CD28- T cells, low T cell proliferative responses in vitro and low IL-2 secretion predicted mortality and together, with increased IL-6 levels and a CD4:CD8 ratio <1, define "Immune Risk Profile" in humans[127]. Based on the above, we decided to find out if some immune functions could be useful as markers of biological age, or "biomarkers," and therefore as predictors of longevity. We felt that this project was worthwhile since biological age is a more adequate parameter than chronological age to measure the rate of aging of a subject, although very seldomly have the proposed batteries of biomarkers included immune functions. Among all functions of immune cells we have focused on the following: a) in lymphocytes, their ability to adhere to the vascular endothelia, migrate towards the site of antigen recognition (chemotaxis), proliferate in response to mitogens and release cytokines such as IL-2; and b) in phagocytes, the process of adherence to tissues, chemotaxis, ingestion or phagocytosis of foreign particles, and destruction of pathogens by means of the intracellular production of free radicals, such as the superoxide anion and other ROS located in the phagosome of these cells. Further, in the NK cells we have analyzed their capacity to destroy tumor cells of the same animal species investigated. The same above parameters have been determined in the various decades of life of human subjects from their twenties to their eighties in leucocytes of peripheral blood, and throughout the life of mice in their peritoneal leucocytes. These types of longitudinal studies, despite their high cost, can be carried out on mice, which have a mean life span of two years but are almost impossible to perform on human subjects. Surprisingly, our results have shown that, in the members of both species, similar age-related changes of the above mentioned immune parameters occur. Thus, with aging there is a decrease of functions such as the lymphoproliferative response and the NK activity that protect us against tumoral cells. There is also a decline of the release of IL-2, as well as a lower chemotaxis capacity, phagocytosis and adequate levels of intracellular ROS, whereas there is an increase of the adherence of immune cells to tissue, which may prevent their arrival to the site where they have to perform their organism-protecting task.

In order to identify the above parameters as markers of biological age and predictors of longevity, we need to demonstrate that the levels they show in a particular subject reveal his real health and senescent conditions. This has been achieved in the following two ways:

a) The first is ascertaining that the individuals with those parameters showing levels older than those of most subjects of the same population, sex and chronological age die before their counterparts. The confirmation that a premature immunosenescence in those parameters may predict a premature death can be tested only in experimental animals. This was performed using a model of premature senescence in mice proposed by our group[24, 25]. The animals that we have denominated PAM (prematurely aging mice), in contrast to the NPAM (non-prematurely aging mice) of the same population, sex and chronological age, are identified by their poor response in a simple T-maze exploration test. This provides strong support for the concept that the nervous and the immune system are closely linked[42]. In mice showing premature aging we have observed that the above mentioned immune functions were performed at the levels characteristic of older mice[26]. In addition to a more significant immunosenescence, the PAM showed high levels of anxiety and a brain neurochemistry characteristic of older animals. Nevertheless, the most convincing evidence that the above mentioned parameters are useful markers of biological age is that the PAM showed a shorter life span than their counterpart NPAM of the same sex and chronological age[25, 26, 42, 117].

b) The additional confirmation of the key role of the immune system in health and longevity is the finding that the subjects reaching a very advanced age preserve the immune functions at levels similar to those of the adults. This has been shown in both humans and experimental animals such as mice. In human subjects our group has ascertained that in healthy centenarians the above mentioned immune functions perform as well as in young-adults (30-year-olds) and much better than in 70-year-old human subjects[101]. A similar finding of a "youthful" conditions has been obtained on peritoneal immune cells of extreme long-lived mice[128].

All the above results confirm that the immune system is a good marker of biological age and a predictor of longevity. Moreover, since the evolution of the mentioned parameters is similar in mice and human subjects, we can assume that men and women showing the above immune parameters at the levels of older subjects have a higher biological age and a shorter longevity.

Chapter 8

The Role of Oxidative Stress and Inflammatory Stress in Immunosenescence

Cells and tissues have developed a sophisticated antioxidant defense system that includes antioxidant defenses, which eventually decompose these potentially injurious oxidizing agents and convert them into harmless derivatives[129]. The enzymatic and nonenzymatic antioxidants are also essential for inhibition of oxidation and inflammation related to the functions of the neutrophils, arachidonic acid and prostaglandin metabolism[130].

The Glutathione Role in the Redox State

It is widely accepted that the glutathione (GSH) is an antioxidant that exerts a critical role on the immune system[131] and many studies have pointed out that GSH depletion is a mainstream in the pathogenesis of several inflammatory/immunomediated diseases. Even if the molecular mechanism underlying this event is still not well known, it might be ascribed to pathways involving the translocation of the nuclear transcription factor kB (NFkB)[132]. The important role exerted by the NFkB in the pathogenesis of several inflammatory/immunomediated diseases is well recognized[133]. Furthermore, the redox status and GSH levels can modulate the immune system in terms of inhibition of IL-1 and T cell receptor-mediated transduction signaling[134]. All these activities act on the regulation of the synthesis of pro-inflammatory cytokines and adhesion molecules, which is impaired in normal conditions, but, most importantly, increases during GSH depletion. Another still unexplored mechanism by which GSH may influence the immune system is by inhibiting the complement system. Therefore, it is conceivable that in subjects affected with chronic inflammatory /immunomediated disorders, low glutathione levels may facilitate complement activation, the trigger/amplification of the inflammatory cascade and, in turn, deposition of complement cleavage fragments on the vascular endothelium[135, 136].

GSH decrease has been associated with aging and the pathogenesis of a variety of diseases, autoimmune or not, including rheumatoid arthritis, autoimmune thyroiditis, muscular dystrophy, amyotrophic lateral sclerosis, AIDS, Alzheimer's disease, alcoholic liver disease, cataract genesis, respiratory distress syndrome, and Werner syndrome[130, 137, 138]. Moreover, high total glutathione concentrations in blood have been related to excellent physical and mental health in women with high longevity[139], and low total glutathione levels in blood have been reported in elderly subjects and patients with chronic diseases[140]. Thus, it has been proposd that aging is cysteine deficiency syndrome[141]. In our studies we observed how total glutathione levels in neutrophils decrease with aging[101, 120].

Why Does Senescence Occur?

To know why immunosenescence occurs, it is necessary to accept that its cause is the same one responsible for the senescence of other cells in the organism, namely the oxidative disorganization linked to the unavoidable use of oxygen to support cellular functions. In addition, as mentioned above, there is a close link between oxidative stress and inflammation, and many of the age-related pathologies are now considered to include in their pathogenesis both oxidative and inflammatory processes[142-148]. In fact, the levels of pro-inflammatory enzymes and molecules, such as cyclooxigenase 2, several cytokines and prostaglandins, increase with age[146]. Moreover, the increase of inflammatory compounds can explain several aspects of immunosenescence[149]. Therefore, aging seems to be associated with an oxidative and inflammatory stress[147, 148].

In trying to answer the question of whether there is increased oxidative and inflammatory stress in the immune cells with aging, our group decided to investigate the age-related changes in the redox and inflammatory state of immune cells. Thus, we have analyzed in immune cells, especially peritoneal leukocytes of mice but also neutrophils and lymphocytes from peripheral blood of humans, a variety of oxidant and inflammatory compounds [extracellular superoxide anion, oxidized glutathione (GSSG), xantin oxidase (XO) activity, TNF-alfa, IL-6, PGE2], and anti-inflammatory and antioxidant protectors, namely IL-10, reduced glutathione (GSH), glutathione peroxidase (GPx), glutathione reductase (GR), superoxide dismutase (SOD) and catalase (CAT), as well as oxidative damage to biomolecules such as lipids and DNA. Our results indicate that with aging leukocytes suffer oxidative and inflammatory stress, resulting in higher levels of the parameters of oxidation and inflammation, decreased antioxidant defense and increased oxidative damage to lipids and DNA[41, 42, 101] (Figure 2). Moreover, increased oxidative and inflammatory stress has also been found in the immune cells of PAM with respect to those of NPAM and in the leukocytes of male mice with respect to those of female mice[42, 117]. In addition, very long-living mice and human centenarians show a redox condition in their immune cells similar to that of healthy adult subjects[101]. In fact, recent studies have pointed out a lower expression of genes resulting in inflammation and oxidation in human centenarians who show preserved immune functions[101, 147, 148]. Thus, centenarians seem to have a peculiar compromise between both pro-inflammatory and anti-inflammatory compounds, and they are remarkably free of most age-related diseases that have an inflammatory component[147, 148]. Although these conditions have not been adequately studied in exceptionally long-living experimental animals, we have observed that peritoneal immune cells from very old mice not only preserve, in general, their function in response to stimuli[128], but also show controlled oxidative-inflammatory stress (data in press).

The age-associated increase of oxidants and inflammatory compounds seems to be related to an up-regulation of a transcription factor as ubiquitous as the nuclear factor-κB (NFκB) activation, which is involved with the expression of genes of oxidant and inflammatory compounds and has been linked to many acute and chronic oxidative and inflammatory disease states[149-153]. Moreover, NFkB is down-regulated by glutathione precursors such as N-acetylcysteine, which prevent excessive oxidation and inflammation in the above situations[151, 152]. Although the activation of NFkB in leucocytes with aging has been scarcely studied, recent articles highlight the role of the NFkB system in aging and immune response[146, 149, 154-156]. Thus, the NFkB binding domain is the genetic regulatory factor most strongly associated with the aging process, and signaling via the longevity factors, such as SIRT1, can inhibit NFkB signaling and simultaneously protect against the inflammaging process[156]. We have analyzed the NFκB activation, in resting conditions, in peritoneal immune cells throughout aging, and our results show that the immune cells from exceptionally long-living mice have levels of activation of NFkB similar to those of younger animals. Moreover, in old mice, only animals with controlled basal NFκB activation in leucocytes achieved high longevity, and the adult animals with a very high activation of the NFkB in their peritoneal leucocytes died early. Thus, the level of activation of NFkB in leucocytes is significantly related to the life expectancy of the subjects from which the cells were obtained (data in press).

The Oxidation-Inflammation Theory of Aging

With all the above results and in agreement with other published data supporting the idea of an inflammation and oxidation condition in aging[146, 157] we have proposed an oxidative-inflammatory theory of aging[40-42]. We suggest that aging is linked to a chronic oxidative stress, which affects all cells of the organism, but especially those of the regulatory systems. Thus, the nervous, endocrine and immune system would show the greatest oxidative damage, being unable to preserve their redox balance. They would suffer functional losses incompatible with an adequate preservation of homeostasis with a resulting increase in morbidity and mortality, such as is found in old age. In addition, the immune system, because of its need to generate continuously oxidative and inflammatory compounds, could activate, if it is not well regulated, factors such as the transcription NFkB, which after reaching certain level of activation, stimulates the expression of genes programming the production of higher amounts of those compounds. Thus, it is likely that if the production of oxidative and inflammatory compounds is not well controlled, the organism may enter in a "vicious cycle" in which the great amount of oxidant and inflammatory compounds produced by the immune system would activate, even more, the further production of the same noxious compounds through factors such as the above mentioned NFkB. If this harmful circle is not well controlled, the noxious compounds in the immune system would disrupt not only the immune cells, but also all other cells of the aging organism (which have a worse response to oxidative stress than young cells), thus contributing to the maintenance of the organism's chronic oxidative stress. In view of all of the above, it seems evident that the immune system can play a role in the uncontrolled oxidation and inflammation process linked to aging and thus affect the speed of aging (Figure 1).

Based on the above, we can say that when an animal shows a great oxidative stress in its immune cells, these have a worse function and that animal shows a decreased longevity. Inversely, if the immune cells of a subject maintain their redox state, their function will be also better, and this subject will reach greater longevity. Thus, there is a relation between the redox state of the immune cells, their functional capacity and the life span of the subject[42](Figure 1). To support this idea and, consequently, the role of the immune system in aging, we can mention experimental models that we have studied and developed as novel approaches to assess premature aging in recent years[40]. We can present two groups with these models: A) Models in which the members of species with high longevity, such as long-lived mice and human centenarians, maintain better immune function and redox state of the immune cells; and B) Models in which the subjects showing an immunosenescence and oxidative and inflammation stress condition, in relation to other members of the group of the same chronological age, as prematurely aging mice (PAM), have a lower life span.

Chapter 9

The Role of the Phagocytic Cells in Oxi-Inflamm-Aging

It is well known that from the time of birth the immune system has to face a great variety of foreign agents, and in order to protect the organism against them, it needs to release toxic oxidants such as reactive oxygen species (ROS) and pro-inflammatory (P-I) compounds. An adequate production of these products, ROS and P-I compounds, is needed to increase the probability that a subject survives to reach the age of reproduction, which is essential for survival of the species. Nevertheless, if ROS and P-I compounds in certain amounts are needed for many physiological processes which are essential for animal survival, then when those amounts are very high, they will lead to oxidative stress and inflammatory stress, respectively. Thus, there are antioxidant (Ax) and anti-inflammatory (An-I) mechanisms to control that excess and the balance between ROS and Ax levels, as well as between P-I and An-I compounds, which are the base of a preserved cellular homeostasis of healthy adulthood (Figure 3). With aging there are more ROS and P-I compounds, as well as less Ax and An-I compounds, available, and the oxidative stress and the inflammatory stress appears. Moreover, oxidation and inflammation are two closely related processes. Thus, with aging the oxi-inflamm-aging, which is the base of the loss of homeostasis, appears (Figure 3). This stress appears since the immune system has not been well prepared to preserve its defensive functions for a long time, especially after the reproductive period. In the case of the members of the human species living in developed countries which show considerable increases in their mean life span, they, in general, suffer the consequences of having a very activated immune system over a long period of time [42, 146, 147, 158, 159]. As it happens with oxygen use, that allows a very active life condition but has as its "side effect" the production of noxious ROS. A very active immune system is designed to provide protection against the risk of contracting infections and tumors to which we are chronically exposed. The counterbalance of the oxygen-inflammation-supported functions and resulting stress is that, if they are not well controlled or the aging organism lacks a satisfactory individual adaptation to this stress, the senescent process accelerates[42]. Thus, the participation of the immune system in the oxi-inflamm-aging seems to be evident, and thus, the immune system can accelerate the aging process andmodulate the biological age and, consequently, the mean longevity.

Based on the above, it seems evident that the leukocytes can play a fundamental role in aging. Moreover, we suggested that this role in the rate of aging is the consequence of the fact that the immune cells produce oxidant and inflammatory compounds in the highest amounts. Even more, with aging, these compounds are produced especially by the phagocytic cells, which are found, with different denominations, in all animals, including the invertebrates[40]. As mentioned above, during aging, adaptive immunity declines, whereas innate immunity, in several aspects, seems to be activated, inducing a pro-inflammatory profile. An evolution-related view of immunosenescence should explain why acquired immunocompetence, which is more specialized and more recent in evolution, is the most impaired with age, whereas the innate immune response (ancestral and less specific) is better preserved and may even be stimulated in excess in the aging organism[155]. In agreement with the above, we have observed that in the peritoneal immune cell populations of mice, as in peripheral blood immune cells of human subjects, the macrophages and neutrophils, respectively, are the immune cells responsible for the generation of higher levels of oxidant compounds than those produced by lymphocytes and these levels significantly increase with age[40, 42]. Thus, it is probable that the phagocytic cells, which are present in all animals, are implicated in the chronic oxidative and inflammatory stress of senescence due to their high age-related increase in the production of oxidants and inflammatory compounds[40-42, 56, 65].

Functions and Redox State in Neutrophils From Centenarians. A Confirmation of the Role of Phagocytic Cells in the Oxi-Inflamm-Aging

Healthy human centenarians represent the best living example of successful aging[160] with well-preserved leukocyte functions[161]. In view of this, we analyzed the most-representative functions of peripheral blood neutrophils in healthy centenarians, according to the SENIEUR protocol, and compared them with those of healthy younger groups: middle-aged and young adults[101]. The results showed better neutrophil functions (adherence, chemotaxis, phagocitosys and superoxide levels) than middle-aged men and women, with levels closer to those of young adult subjects. The neutrophils of centenarians maintained all the above functions to an extent similar to young adult subjects and better than the middle-aged group. This better immune condition could contribute to extreme longevity. Interestingly, previous studies of neutrophil function in centenarians revealed that phagocytic ability was increased, whereas superoxide generation was decreased compared to middle-aged subjects[162]. These data suggest that maintenance of neutrophil phagocytic capacity is important for longevity, and it can overcome the age-related decline in superoxide-generating ability. Moreover, when the functions of phagocytic cells are better in old mice, the longevity of the animals increases[117].

Regarding the redox state, for antioxidant parameters, peripheral blood neutrophils from centenarians showed levels of glutathione and catalase activity, two important antioxidant parameters that are closely related to longevity, similar to those of adult subjects[43]. Lower levels of reactive oxygen species have been reported in longer-living strains of houseflies and mice[121, 122]. High total glutathione concentrations in blood have been related to excellent physical and mental health in longevous women[139]. Regarding catalase activity, neutrophils from centenarians show the highest antioxidant enzyme activity. Some studies have found a relationship between catalase activity and higher longevity[163], which could be related to the important role this enzyme plays in tolerance to oxidative stress and adaptive cell response (because it acts only in the presence of high levels of $H2O2$). There are reports of a plasmatic antioxidant status maintained in people aged 90 and older at a level similar to that of the control population (23–66 years)[164]; therefore, the antioxidant status shown by centenarians could be an important advantage in avoiding altered age-associated redox status.

The centenarians studied had well-preserved antioxidant ability, low superoxide anion production, and no altered peripheral blood neutrophil functions. Therefore, these characteristics could be goals that would enable them to avoid age-associated diseases and attain longevity. The oxidative stress of the immune cells seems to be the basis of their functional deterioration with aging[41, 117]. In agreement with the oxidant–inflammatory theory of aging, it is possible that the better redox state of neutrophils in centenarians helps them to achieve a better health and to prevent the age-related diseases. The results could provide further evidence of the usefulness of these determinations as markers of ''biological age'' and, therefore, predictors of survival in humans.

Chapter 10

Influential Factors over the Functional and Redox Parameters in Neutrophils

There are several kinds of factors that can modulate the functions and the redox state in leukocytes, in general, and in phagocytic cells, in particular. In the present section we are going to comment on only two of these factors: gender differences and the circadian and seasonal rhythms.

Gender Differences

In the mammalian species, females usually have better immune functions than males[165]. Moreover, females also have a longer mean life span owing to the effects of the estrogens that allow them to live in a less oxidized condition[166]. In fact, recent studies report that the greater longevity of mammalian females, including humans, is associated with better antioxidant capacity[166, 167], which has been observed in the mitochondria, and it could be associated with circulating estrogen levels, because estrogen is able to improve antioxidant capacity[168]. This better redox state in females seems to be reflected in the better redox state of their leucocytes (data in press). Thus, we have observed in mice this different life expectancy and a better immune function in females than males, in both rats and mice.

Table 1. Several function and oxidation parameters in peritoneal macrophages from female and male adult (20 weeks of age) ICR (CD1) mice. Mean and maximum life span in these groups

Parameters	Females	Males
Adherence Index (%)	26±4	48±12**
Chemotaxis Index (no. of cells on filter)	822±115	634±79**
Phagocytososis Index (No. particles/100 cells)	251±41	275±36
Intracellular Superoxide Anion (nmols/10^6 cells)	51±12	44±11
Extracell. Superoxide Anion (nmols/10^6 cells)	17±6	22±3*
Mean life span (weeks)	87.5	75.8
Maximum life span in these groups (weeks)	121	108

*P< 0.05: **P<0.01 with respect to the corresponding value in females.

The scarce results in this context are focused on lymphocyte functions[165], but there are no results in phagocytic cells such as macrophages.

In Table 1 we show differences in several functions of peritoneal macrophages from adult female and male ICR (CD1) mice. The chemotaxis capacity of macrophages was significantly increase in females with respect to males of the same chronological age, whereas the adherence capacity and the extracellular superoxide anion levels, two parameters that increase with age, were smaller in females than males. Although the phagocytic index (number of particles of latex ingested by 100 macrophages) is similar in females and males, we have data from adult BALB/c mice in which this index was higher (P<0.01) in females than in males (479±41 and 324±60, respectively). Moreover, those females showed a higher mean longevity than males, as well as a higher maximum longevity in females than in males.

In the neutrophil functions, when we compared the mentioned parameters between men and women at different chronological ages, we did not find differences between young adult men and women[66], but in elderly men the values of superoxide anion were significantly higher than in women. In other study[101] the only difference observed was that young adult women had significantly lower levels of superoxide anions than young adult men. This difference was lost when they became elderly, showing a trend toward higher levels in middle-aged women. Other authors have observed that the neutrophils from adult women have a similar phagocytosis index with latex particles to men. However, those neutrophils of women showed a significant increase in the phagocytosis of candida albicans and in the microbicide capacity of these yeasts than those of men[169]. These results seem to indicate that depending on the concrete type of capacity measured, the method used, the age, or the group of subjects, the results can be different in the phagocytic cell function comparison between females and males.

Although no significant differences were found between centenarian men and women, men had better values than women in all the neutrophil functions studied[101]. Sex differences in the health status of centenarians have been reported, indicating that centenarian men are less heterogeneous and healthier than centenarian women. Because mean longevity in men is lower than in women, men who reach very old age represent a survival collective in better condition than women of the same age. Immunological factors regarding the age-related increase in pro-inflammatory status and the frequency of human leukocyte antigen ancestral haplotypes also show sex differences that probably contribute to the difference in longevity between men and women[170].

Circadian and Annual Seasonal Rhythms

The cyclic changes that occur in physiological processes are known as biological rhythms. These biological oscillations have different frequencies, and they are due to the need to anticipate the periodic and predictable changes of the environment. The biological rhythms are genetically coded because of their endogenous origin, even though they may be adjusted to the periodic surroundings by ambient time cues, referred to as environmental synchronizers or entraining agents (light, temperature, light-dark cycle, seasonal changes, etc)[171].

The biological oscillations can be denominated according to their timing and length. For instance, those which last 24 hours are known as circadian rhythms and are kept in step with the daily light span. In addition, the rhythms with a period of about 1 year, or seasonal variations, are observed under different climatic conditions suggesting they are manifestations of an endogenous biological clock[172].

Virtually all neuroendocrine and immunological parameters investigated in different experimental animals and humans display biological periodicity, showing an intricate time structure with rhythms and pulsate variations in multiple frequencies[172]. Circadian rhythm is revealed for every hormone in circulation, as well as for circulating immune cells, lymphocyte metabolism and transformability, cytokines, receptors and adhesion molecules[173]. Regarding the immune system, and specifically phagocytic function, several studies support the idea that this system experiments with both circadian and seasonal rhythms[174, 175].

Nowadays it is accepted that the pineal gland becomes a principal organ involved in the control of rhythmic adaptations to daily and seasonal cycles in mammals. Therefore, the hormone that this gland produces, melatonin, acts as a circadian clock, giving a time-related signal to a number of body functions, such as the immune response[176]. Moreover, the immunomodulatory and antioxidant role of melatonin has been assumed in recent years, and it has been shown to be involved in the regulation of both cellular and humoral immunity[177]. Several experiments have shown a direct action of melatonin on the phagocytic process. Thus, both phagocytic index and efficiency are enhanced during the dark period, being positively correlated with melatonin serum levels. However, superoxide anion levels are decreased and are negatively correlated with the levels of melatonin[174]. Moreover, the regulatory function of melatonin on immune response is seasonally dependent. This fact may account for the cyclic pattern of symptom expression shown by certain infectious diseases, which become more pronounced at particular seasons of the year[177].

The decrease of melatonin production with aging[178] contributes to the decline in immune function[179]. Thus, some studies show an altered secretion pattern of melatonin with aging and an enhancing effect of the hormone on phagocytic function of young animals with respect to the aged group[175]. Several studies have demonstrated that exogenous melatonin, as well as tryptophan administration, increases phagocytosis and free-radical scavenging in both young and old animals[179]. Therefore, melatonin has the potential therapeutic value of enhancing immune function in aged individuals[180]. Recently, we have carried out a study on the phagocytic functions of neutrophils at two different times of day (Table 2), as well as on the different seasons of year, through human aging (Figure 4). In Table 2 the results of several neutrophil function parameters in cells from young adult men and women obtained at 10 h and at 15 h are shown. We can see a smaller spontaneous mobility, chemotaxis and basal levels of intracellular superoxide anion in neutrophils at 15 h with respect to these values at 10 h. Thus, at 15 h the functional capacity of neutrophils could be less effective than at 10h.

Table 2. Several parameters of neutrophil functions in blood cells obtained at 10h and 15 h from a group of young adult men and women

Parameters	10h	15h
Adherence Index (%)	34±7	32±7
Spontaneous Mobility Index (no. cells per filter)	339±59	244±17*
Chemotaxis Index (no. cells per filter)	357±44	257±26*
Phagocytosis Index (no. particles ingested per 100 cells)	845±41	828±72
Intracellular Superoxide Anion (Basal levels)(nmols/10^6 cells)	40±4	31±2**
Intracellular Superoxide Anion Stimulation Index (%)	43±9	49±8
Parameters	10h	15h

*$P<0.05$; **$P<0.01$ with respect to the corresponding value at 10 h.

One possible reason would be the lower levels of melatonin with the advancing day, but other factors submitted to circadian variations can also be involved.

With respect to the seasonal changes (Figure 4), we have observed how summer and winter are the seasons in which the functions of neutrophils are most affected, especially in mature and elderly men and women, in agreement with the fact that it is in these seasons when the number of infectious processes increase in older people.

The study of the structural and temporal pattern of the immune system would allow the development of new techniques for diagnosis, prognosis, therapy and assessment of risk factors in immunopathological conditions.

Chapter 11

Neutrophils and their Roles in Disease

Immunosenescence, as the result of direct or indirect changes to both the innate and adaptive immune systems, has numerous and varied clinical consequences. The links between aging, immunosenescence, and diseases associated with inflammatory conditions have recently received great attention. Increased morbidity and mortality related to bacterial and viral infection[5-8], decreased vaccine effectiveness[8,181-184], increased incidence of autoimmune disease such as diabetes, rheumatoid arthritis, and systemic lupus erythematosus[185,186], inflammation-associated diseases including neurodegenerative diseases such as Alzheimer's disease and Parkinson's disease[187], age-related macular degeneration[188], related inflammatory conditions[185-187, 189, 190] and increased incidence of cancer[186, 191, 192] have been associated with immunosenescence. Elevated serum pro-inflammatory cytokines have been associated with an increased risk of heart disease, high blood pressure, type 2 diabetes, and atherosclerosis[193-196].

Moreover, aged people are more likely to acquire chronic infections and this virological status impacts on immunity. Chronic infection by some of these pathogens (Epstein-Barr virus, Cytomegalovirus...) may alter the immune system and lead to consequences (immunosenescence) similar to those induced by aging directly[197, 198]. Because of this, the ability to mount a vigorous immune response is essential for survival in infectious environments, but the long-term consequences of the associated unintended damage can be severe. Several studies have observed that a genetic predisposition to weak inflammatory activity (for example high IL-10 or low tumor necrosis factor-α) is beneficial for longevity, provided individuals escape succumbing to infection[199, 200]. In other words, as long as these individuals live within a microbially nonhazardous environment, a weak inflammatory response will be beneficial in counteracting frequent diseases of the aged, such as dementia and cardiovascular disease.

The chronic low-grade inflammatory state associated with aging is clearly shown by the increase in serum levels of inflammatory mediators. A wide range of factors have been claimed to contribute to this state, although chronic antigenic stress, which affects the immune system throughout life with a progressive activation of phagocytic cells, seems to play one of the most important roles[41, 158]. This pro-inflammatory status, known as "inflamm-aging"[158], which interacts with the genetic background, has the potential to trigger the onset of age-related inflammatory diseases, such as atherosclerosis[170] and other conditions. The "inflamm-aging" network has been used to guide an understanding of the aetiology of inflammation in the diseases of old age, and a particularly valuable resource has been genetic studies in successfully aging populations[186, 199, 201, 202]. It has been proposed that the increase in life expectancy at older ages over history might not only be due to improvements in sanitation and medical care, but also be related to reduced inflammation during early life, leading to increases in morbidity and mortality due to chronic conditions in old age[203]. The implications are a potential slowing of lifespan extension in developed countries but a welcome expectation that longevity will increase with the recent fall in child infection rates in developing countries[204].

Chapter 12

Strategies to Revitalize the Neutrophil Functions in Aging

Diet. Role of Antioxidants in the Neutrophil Function and Redox State

Currently the existence of an oxidant-antioxidant imbalance in aging is accepted. The first observations suggesting a key role for oxidative injury in aging were those showing the favorable effects of endogenous and dietary antioxidants, which have been demonstrated in experimental animals and human subjects[40, 205]. A direct link between oxidative stress, aging and human diseases can be further established by studies analyzing the impact of variation in human genes encoded for antioxidant defense systems[206]. Moreover, the endogenous antioxidants decrease in oxidative stress situations, such as endotoxemia and aging, because they are spent neutralizing the excess of ROS[41, 42, 152, 205]. Thus, it is generally accepted that biological age and mean longevity may be associated with an optimal antioxidant protection. Moreover, the senescent decrease in antioxidant levels supports the free radical theory of aging and provides a rationale for attempts to decrease the rate of aging by supplementing the diet with antioxidants[41, 42, 81, 205].

The ingestion of a diet enriched with antioxidants seems to be adequate for maintaining an optimum redox balance and therefore protecting the aging organism against oxygen stress. Thus, the administration of compounds such as vitamins C and E, polyphenols and thiolic antioxidants such as taurine, thioproline (TP) and N-acetylcisteine (NAC), among others, which are precursors of reduced glutathione (GSH), in isolation or in nutritional formulations containing several compounds, may be recommended, because of their antioxidant and anti-inflammmatory action. In fact, previous studies performed in our laboratory in chronologically-old mice, in PAM and in elderly men and women have demonstrated the beneficial effect of those antioxidants, which show important favorable effects on health, acting on the nervous and the immune systems[40-42, 65, 81, 120, 205, 207-220]. We have observed that supplementation of diet with those antioxidants improves the immune function in aging mice, bringing it to adult values. Even more, it neutralizes the oxidative stress, helping to reach values of oxidants, antioxidants and biomolecular damage similar to those of adults and NPAM in mice, and adults in humans[40]. These results have been obtained in mouse peritoneal macrophages and in human blood neutrophils (Figure 2). In neutrophils from elderly men and women we have observed the favorable effect of the ingestion of vitamin E66, Vitamin C (unpublished data) and NAC120.

As it has been mentioned above, the performance of the leukocytes' function may exhaust their reserves of antioxidants[221]. This could help to explain why in laboratory animals and human subjects the homeostasis-linked functional competence of the immune system in the adult age is improved after diet supplementation with appropriate amounts of antioxidants such as vitamin C, vitamin E, thiol antioxidants and polyphenols[215, 222-224].

Since the favorable action of the antioxidants on the immune system is expressed as an increase of the functions that are depressed and a decrease of those that are excessively active, the antioxidants cannot be considered general immunostimulants. In fact, they may bring each immune function and redox state to its optimum, thus acting as immunomodulators. This modulating ability appears to be focused at the level of the ubiquitous intracellular factors implicated in oxidation and inflammation, such as the NFkB[152].

It is accepted that the antioxidants play a role in the recovery of a great number of nervous functions[225]. Thus, the regulatory role of the antioxidants would be performed not only on the immune system, but also on the other regulatory systems, including the nervous system, in which the oxidative stress also underlies its senescent impairment. Moreover, in the PAM the ingestion of thiolic antioxidants not only improves the immune function, but also the behavioral response[117, 207].

Even more interestingly, this immune "rejuvenation", as well as the improvement of the nervous system, in the laboratory mice is accompanied by a greater longevity[41].

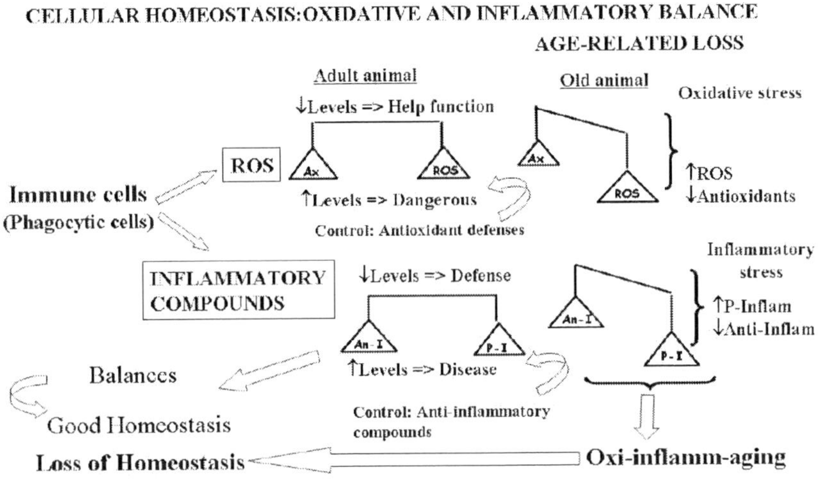

CELLULAR HOMEOSTASIS: OXIDATIVE AND INFLAMMATORY BALANCE AGE-RELATED LOSS

Figure 2. The phagocytes are involved in the oxidative and inflammatory balance that supports cellular homeostasis. The phagocytic cells produce oxidants, especially reactive oxygen species (ROS) and inflammatory compounds in their defensive work against pathogens. These compounds, in certain amounts, are needed for the appropriate defensive function of these cells. However, when the amounts of ROS and inflammatory compounds are very high, and they overcome the antioxidant and anti-inflammatory defenses, an oxidative and inflammatory stress appears (an imbalance with greater oxidants and inflammatory compounds than antioxidants and anti-inflammatory compounds). The adequate function of phagocytic cells and of the organism is based on a perfect balance between the levels of ROS and those of antioxidants, as well as the balance between the levels of inflammatory and anti-inflammatory compounds, which occurs in healthy adults. The losses of these balances that occur with age produce oxidative and inflammatory stress, increasing the oxi-inflamm-aging situation, which is the basis of the loss of homeostasis.

We have also found (unpublished work) that chronologically old mice and PAM with an antioxidant supplemented diet (mixes of antioxidants, such as vitamin C, vitamin E, b-carotene, zinc and selenium, in very little amounts, and TP and NAC) show a significant increase in their life span.

According to a recent review, antioxidants, such as NAC and alpha-lipoic acid, are able to neutralize free radicals at their sites of production in the mitochondria, and although they are unable to increase the species-characteristic maximum life span, they may increase mean individual longevity[205].

In humans, the results obtained after supplementation on the immune system are due to a decrease of the oxidative stress in these cells, in a similar way to those observed in leukocytes from mice. Since the improvements in the immune functions found with antioxidant supplementation are similar in humans and mice, and because these changes in mice are accompanied by an increase in the life span, it is probable that similar effects could be obtained in humans.

Physical Exercise

Physical activity is deemed to have a beneficial effect on health, and it has been associated with having less susceptibility to infections and other pathologies compared to sedentary people. Because of this, the performance of physical activity is another lifestyle factor that can improve health and quality of life in old subjects[226]. There is a wealth of information on the effects of physical exercise on the immune function of adult, experimental animals and humans. Although conflicting results have been obtained, depending on the type of exercise, immune function studied or state of the subject, it is generally accepted that an acute or very strong training induces an inflammatory response with selective activation or depression of immune cell functions, whereas moderate training exercise leads to clear benefits of the immune system with improvement of their functions[227]. However, recent studies have shown that this general finding cannot be extended to the innate immune response and, particularly, to phagocytes. Thus, some stages of the phagocytic process are stimulated by both moderate and intense exercise in both experimental animals[228] and humans[229]. However, the profile of pro-/anti-inflammatory cytokine release seems to be better following the moderate exercise[229].

It is accepted that physical exercise is a stress and, in most of cases, both exercise and stress, are indistinguishable at levels of nervous and hormonal mediators. For this reason, the effects of exercise on the immune response are mediated by stress hormones and factors[230]. However, in this context the general statement that stress induces immunosuppression cannot be assumed at all levels of the immune system. In fact, although those stress factors can impair some specific immune functions, they may also stimulate different aspects of the innate immune and inflammatory response[230]. Thus, phagocytes seem to play a major role in the defense against infection during exercise-induced stress, and this is probably useful in preventing the entry and maintenance of microorganisms where the specific response seems to be depressed. Thus, recently we have reviewed the exercise-induced neuroimmunomodulation and the role of catecholamines as "stress mediators" and/or "danger signals" for the innate immune response during physical exercise[231].

In addition, strenuous physical exercise may be a significant oxidative stress because it increases consumption of molecular oxygen for respiration and may generate higher amounts of ROS. According to several reviews, vigorous exercise is accompanied by the involvement of immune cells, especially phagocytic cells, in the generation of oxidants[232] through the activation of factors such as NFkB[233]. Thus, an over-stimulation of the innate immune response could be harmful for those subjects with a high inflammatory state. However, a well controlled and regulated stimulation of the innate immune mechanisms during moderate exercise can help to prevent infections and, as has been reviewed by Johnson[234], in response to repetitive or graded exercise training, a decrease in oxidative stress and a resistance to oxidative damage appears. This fact may be due to exercise-induced changes in antioxidant enzymes not only in the skeletal muscle, which is recognized as a major source of free radical generation, but also in other tissues and cells. Although the results show discrepancies depending on the species, tissue, type and subtype of cell, age of the animal and training regimen, in general an up-regulation of antioxidant defenses appears with moderate exercise training[234]. With regard to the immune cells, the downregulation of the release of ROS and the adaptation of antioxidant mechanisms to regular exercise has been observed in phagocytic cells by us and other authors[233, 235].

Although in old animals or elderly humans the effects of physical exercise on the immune functions have been scarcely studied, the available data show that the practice of moderate exercise is an important candidate for improving the immune function in the elderly. In fact, several authors and our own group have shown that, in old animals, regular exercise training improves immune functions[103, 227]. In addition, we have observed that the favorable effects of exercise are higher in old mice than in young mice[103] and similar results have been revealed in humans[41]. We have observed that elderly men and women who performed moderate physical exercise for 6 months (3 sessions of 45 minutes per week), significantly improved their immune system with regard to neutrophil, lymphocyte and NK functions, bringing the values close to those in adults[41].

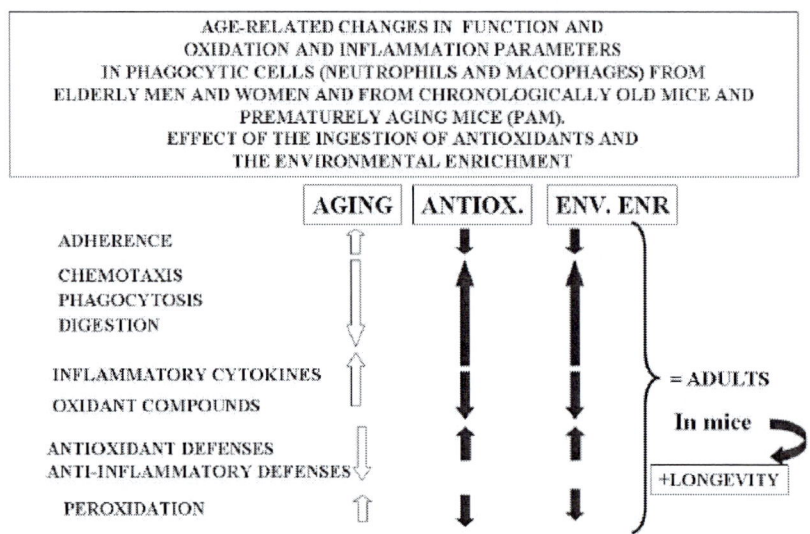

Figure 3. Age-related changes in function, oxidation and inflammatory parameters of phagocytic cells from humans and mice. Role of antioxidants and environmental enrichment on these parameters and on the longevity of mice. With aging, there are changes in several parameters of function (increased the adherence at tissue but decreased the chemotaxis, the phagocytosis and the digestion capacity), redox (increased the oxidant compound levels and decreased the antioxidant capacity) and inflammation (increased the inflammatory compounds and decreased the anti-inflammatory compounds) states in phagocytic cells from humans and mice. These parameters are modulated by the ingestion of appropriate amounts of antioxidants and by an environmental enrichment that bring the values of these parameters, in elderly humans and in chronologically old or prematurely aging experimental animals, closer to those in the corresponding adult subjects or non-prematurely aging controls. In mice, the animals ingesting antioxidants in the diet and with environmental enrichment show an increase in their longevity. ANTIOX: antioxidants; ENV. ENR: environmental enrichment.

It is possible that the effect of physical exercise, improving the immune cell functions, is carried out directly on these cells through the factors released in response to exercise and through an increase of their above mentioned antioxidant defenses[41, 234]. In fact, we found that the increases in ascorbate content in macrophages after exercise in both young and old mice[235] and in humans after a moderate physical exercise, not only improves several functions of peripheral blood neutrophils and lymphocytes, but also increases their antioxidant defenses[41]. Moreover, the production of pro-inflammatory and anti-inflammatory cytokines decreases and increases, respectively, after moderate physical exercise[229, 236], and the inflammatory markers are lower in older adults performing exercise than in those without physical activity[237]. Thus, moderate physical exercise could decrease the rate of aging by recovering the oxidant/antioxidant balance of the immune cells [41] and decrease the inflamm-aging.

Other Factors of Lifestyle

Other intervention systems for decreasing the rate of aging that we are studying are the mental activity, as well as overcoming of emotional stress. Thus, our preliminary results have shown that mice with environmental enrichment show an improvement of the functions and redox state of their immune cells[238]. Moreover, a recent work (unpublished data) with mice confirms the importance of maintaining active mental and/or physical activity, obtained through that environmental enrichment, to improve quality of life in terms of immunity, and concretely in phagocytic functions, demonstrates that this active life must be initiated at the early stages of the aging process and preserved until death to improve life span (Figure 3).

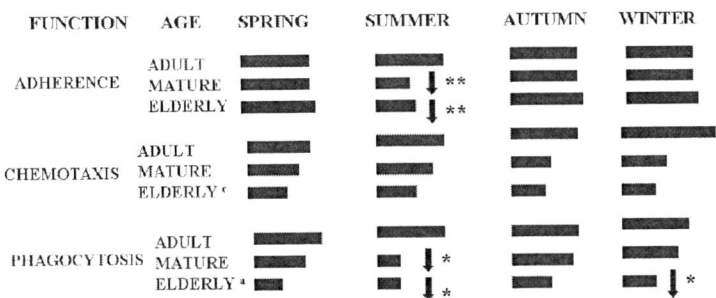

Figure 4. Seasonal and age-related changes in several human neutrophil functions. In summer and winter the values of functions of neutrophils are decreased in mature and elderly men and women in comparison to those in the other seasons. *p<0.05; **p<0.01 with respect to the other seasons. a:p<0.05; c: p<0.001 with respect to the adult values.

Chapter 13

Conclusion

Aging affects many components of the organism and supposes a reduction of the homeostasis, the adaptive capacity and a loss of response capacity to changes. This loss of homeostasis affects the immune system, which is an excellent marker of health[20]. Several studies have analyzed the age-related changes in the innate and adaptive immune systems. According to the role of oxidative stress and inflammatory stress in immunosenesce and according to several studies performed in animal models and humans, we can suggest that the neutrophil dysfunction and the imbalance between pro-oxidants and antioxidants in the neutrophils of aged individuals can be assumed to trigger of the aging process. Even more, the altered functional parameters and redox imbalance seem to be excellent markers of biological age and longevity. Thus, we could say that when an animal shows a great oxidative stress in its immune cells, these have a worse function and a decreased longevity[117]. Inversely, if the immune cells of a subject maintain their redox state, their function will also be better and this subject will reach greater longevity[117, 128]. In analyzing the redox state in healthy centenarians, the best example of successful aging, these parameters are lower than in cells from middle-aged subjects. Moreover, if the oxidative stress of the immune cells is the basis of their functional deterioration with aging[41], it seems evident that the redox state of neutrophils in centenarians enables them to function better and, therefore, to avoid age-related diseases. Moreover, the better function and redox state shown by the neutrophils of centenarians with respect to of middle-aged subjects supports the oxidant-inflammatory theory of aging[41]. Different studies have been performed to modify the redox state of the organism, and supplementation with appropriate amount of antioxidants in elderly men and women, as well as the administration of diet with these antioxidants to old mice, seem to improve the neutrophils' and macrophage functions, respectively, and bring the values of their functions to those found in adult subjects[40, 41], [66, 81]. Similar results have been obtained with other strategies of lifestyle, such as performed physical exercise or a good control of stress[41]. We could suggest the function parameters studied in neutrophils as biomarkers of "biological age" and predictors of survival. Although this opens a door to look for new ways to improve the immune function, and thus life span, further studies are needed to confirm these ideas and better understand the immune basis of the privileged aging process of centenarians.

Acknowledgments

The authors would like to thank Dr. Miquel for his critical revision of the article and also express their gratitude to Dr. Arranz, Dr. Guayerbas and Mr. Carpintero for their invaluable help in performing the experiments which have allowed the authors to arrive at some of the ideas expressed in this article. This work was supported by grants of the MCINN (BFU2008-04336), Research Group of UCM (910379ENEROINN) and RETICEF (RD06/0013/0003) (ISCIII).

References

[1] Borkan GA, Norris AH. Assessment of biological age using a profile of physical parameters. *J. Gerontol.* Mar 1980;35(2):177-184.

[2] Borkan GA, Norris AH. Biological age in adulthood: comparison of active and inactive U.S. males. *Hum Biol.* Dec 1980;52(4):787-802.

[3] Makinodan T, Kay MM. Age influence on the immune system. *Adv. Immunol.* 1980;29:287-330.

[4] Murasko DM, Nelson BJ, Silver R, Matour D, Kaye D. Immunologic response in an elderly population with a mean age of 85. *Am. J. Med.* Oct 1986;81(4):612-618.

[5] Bender BS. Infectious disease risk in the elderly. *Immunol. Allergy Clin North Am.* Feb 2003;23(1):57-64, vi.

[6] Falsey AR, Walsh EE. Respiratory syncytial virus infection in elderly adults. *Drugs Aging.* 2005;22(7):577-587.

[7] High KP, Bradley S, Loeb M, Palmer R, Quagliarello V, Yoshikawa T. A new paradigm for clinical investigation of infectious syndromes in older adults: assessment of functional status as a risk factor and outcome measure. *Clin. Infect. Dis.* Jan 1 2005;40(1):114-122.

[8] Nichol KL. Influenza vaccination in the elderly: impact on hospitalisation and mortality. *Drugs Aging.* 2005;22(6):495-515.

[9] O'Meara ES, White M, Siscovick DS, Lyles MF, Kuller LH. Hospitalization for pneumonia in the Cardiovascular Health Study: incidence, mortality, and influence on longer-term survival. *J. Am. Geriatr. Soc.* Jul 2005;53(7):1108-1116.

[10] Franceschi C, Monti D, Barbieri D, et al. Immunosenescence in humans: deterioration or remodelling? *Int. Rev. Immunol.* 1995;12(1):57-74.

[11] Miller RA. The aging immune system: primer and prospectus. *Science.* Jul 5 1996;273(5271):70-74.

[12] Pawelec G, Effros RB, Caruso C, Remarque E, Barnett Y, Solana R. T cells and aging (update february 1999). *Front Biosci.* Mar 1 1999;4:D216-269.

[13] Effros RB. Ageing and the immune system. *Novartis Found Symp.* 2001;235:130-139; discussion 139-145, 146-139.

[14] Kohut ML, Senchina DS. Reversing age-associated immunosenescence via exercise. *Exerc. Immunol Rev.* 2004;10:6-41.

[15] Strehler BL. Time, cells and aging. *New York: Academic Press-* 1977.

[16] Kirkwood TB, Feder M, Finch CE, et al. What accounts for the wide variation in life span of genetically identical organisms reared in a constant environment? *Mech. Ageing Dev.* Mar 2005;126(3):439-443.

[17] Sander M, Avlund K, Lauritzen M, et al. Aging-from molecules to populations. *Mech. Ageing Dev.* Oct 2008;129(10):614-623.

[18] Finkel D, Whitfield K, McGue M. Genetic and environmental influences on functional age: a twin study. *J. Gerontol. B Psychol. Sci. Soc. Sci.* Mar 1995;50(2):P104-113.

[19] Bae CY, Kang YG, Kim S, et al. Development of models for predicting biological age (BA) with physical, biochemical, and hormonal parameters. *Arch. Gerontol. Geriatr.* Sep-Oct 2008;47(2):253-265.

[20] Wayne SJ, Rhyne RL, Garry PJ, Goodwin JS. Cell-mediated immunity as a predictor of morbidity and mortality in subjects over 60. *J. Gerontol.* Mar 1990;45(2):M45-48.

[21] Ferguson FG, Wikby A, Maxson P, Olsson J, Johansson B. Immune parameters in a longitudinal study of a very old population of Swedish people: a comparison between survivors and nonsurvivors. *J. Gerontol. A Biol. Sci .Med. Sci.* Nov 1995;50(6):B378-382.

[22] Ma YX, Yue Z, Wang ZS, et al. Physiological basis for long life span. *Mech. Ageing Dev.* Oct 1997;98(1):47-55.

[23] Ogata K, Yokose N, Tamura H, et al. Natural killer cells in the late decades of human life. *Clin. Immunol. Immunopathol.* Sep 1997;84(3):269-275.

[24] Guayerbas N, Puerto M, Victor VM, Miquel J, De la Fuente M. Leukocyte function and life span in a murine model of premature immunosenescence. *Exp. Gerontol.* Jan-Mar 2002;37(2-3):249-256.

[25] Guayerbas N, Catalan M, Victor VM, Miquel J, De la Fuente M. Relation of behaviour and macrophage function to life span in a murine

model of premature immunosenescence. *Behav. Brain. Res.* Aug 21 2002;134(1-2):41-48.

[26] Guayerbas N, De La Fuente M. An impairment of phagocytic function is linked to a shorter life span in two strains of prematurely aging mice. *Dev. Comp. Immunol.* Apr 2003;27(4):339-350.

[27] Medvedev ZA. An attempt at a rational classification of theories of ageing. *Biol. Rev. Camb. Philos. Soc.* Aug 1990;65(3):375-398.

[28] Carnes BA, Staats DO, Sonntag WE. Does senescence give rise to disease? *Mech Ageing Dev.* Dec 2008;129(12):693-699.

[29] Vina J, Borras C, Miquel J. Theories of ageing. *IUBMB Life.* Apr-May 2007;59(4-5):249-254.

[30] Hayflick L. The Limited in Vitro Lifetime of Human Diploid Cell Strains. *Exp. Cell Res.* Mar 1965;37:614-636.

[31] Goyns MH. Genes, telomeres and mammalian ageing. *Mech. Ageing Dev.* Apr 2002;123(7):791-799.

[32] Pearl R. The rate of living. *London: University of London Press.* 1928.

[33] Weissman A. Essays upon heredity and kindred biological problems. *London-New York: Oxford University Press-Clarendon.* 1891.

[34] Hayflick L. Biological aging is no longer an unsolved problem. *Ann. N Y Acad .Sci.* Apr 2007;1100:1-13.

[35] Miquel J, Economos AC, Fleming J, Johnson JE, Jr. Mitochondrial role in cell aging. *Exp. Gerontol.* 1980;15(6):575-591.

[36] Harman D. Aging: a theory based on free radical and radiation chemistry. *J Gerontol.* Jul 1956;11(3):298-300.

[37] Harman D. The biologic clock: the mitochondria? *J. Am. Geriatr. Soc.* Apr 1972;20(4):145-147.

[38] Miquel J. An integrated theory of aging as the result of mitochondrial-DNA mutation in differentiated cells. *Arch Gerontol Geriatr.* Mar-Jun 1991;12(2-3):99-117.

[39] Williams GC. Pleiotropy, natural selection and the evolution of senescence. *Evolution.* 1957;2:397-411.

[40] De la Fuente M, Miquel J. An update of the oxidation-inflammation theory of aging: the involvement of the immune system in oxi-inflamm-aging. *Curr. Pharm. Des.* 2009;15(26):3003-3026.

[41] De la Fuente M, Hernanz A, Vallejo MC. The immune system in the oxidative stress conditions of aging and hypertension: favorable effects of antioxidants and physical exercise. *Antioxid Redox Signal.* Sep-Oct 2005;7(9-10):1356-1366.

[42] De la Fuente M. Role of neuroimmunomodulation in aging. *Neuroimmunomodulation.* 2008;15(4-6):213-223.
[43] De la Fuente M. The immune system as a marker of health and
[44] longevity. . *Antiaging Med.* 2004;1:31-41.
[45] Besedovsky HO, del Rey A. Immune-neuro-endocrine interactions: facts and hypotheses. *Endocr. Rev.* Feb 1996;17(1):64-102.
[46] Wrona D. Neural-immune interactions: an integrative view of the bidirectional relationship between the brain and immune systems. *J. Neuroimmunol.* Mar 2006;172(1-2):38-58.
[47] Besedovsky HO, Rey AD. Physiology of psychoneuroimmunology: a personal view. *Brain Behav Immun.* Jan 2007;21(1):34-44.
[48] Blalock JE. The immune system as a sensory organ. *J. Immunol.* Mar 1984;132(3):1067-1070.
[49] Arranz L, Guayerbas N, De la Fuente M. Impairment of several immune functions in anxious women. *J .Psychosom. Res.* Jan 2007;62(1):1-8.
[50] Arranz L, de Vicente A, Munoz M, De la Fuente M. Impaired immune function in a homeless population with stress-related disorders. *Neuroimmunomodulation.* 2009;16(4):251-260.
[51] Barak Y. The immune system and happiness. *Autoimmun. Rev.* Oct 2006;5(8):523-527.
[52] Merril JE. *Production and influence of inflammatory cytokines in diseases of the adult central nervous system.* San Diego: Academic Press; 2001.
[53] Smith RG, Betancourt L, Sun Y. Molecular endocrinology and physiology of the aging central nervous system. *Endocr. Rev.* Apr 2005;26(2):203-250.
[54] Fabris N. A neuroendocrine-immune theory of aging. *Int. J. Neurosci.* Apr 1990;51(3-4):373-375.
[55] High KP. Infection as a cause of age-related morbidity and mortality. *Ageing Res Rev.* Jan 2004;3(1):1-14.
[56] Ortega E, Garcia JJ, De La Fuente M. Ageing modulates some aspects of the non-specific immune response of murine macrophages and lymphocytes. *Exp. Physiol.* Sep 2000;85(5):519-525.
[57] Sebastian C, Espia M, Serra M, Celada A, Lloberas J. MacrophAging: a cellular and molecular review. *Immunobiology.* 2005;210(2-4):121-126.
[58] Gruver AL, Hudson LL, Sempowski GD. Immunosenescence of ageing. *J. Pathol.* Jan 2007;211(2):144-156.
[59] Aw D, Silva AB, Palmer DB. Immunosenescence: emerging challenges for an ageing population. *Immunology.* Apr 2007;120(4):435-446.

[60] Kumar R, Burns EA. Age-related decline in immunity: implications for vaccine responsiveness. *Expert Rev Vaccines.* May 2008;7(4):467-479.

[61] Pawelec G, Barnett Y, Forsey R, et al. T cells and aging, January 2002 update. *Front. Biosci.* May 1 2002;7:d1056-1183.

[62] Gregg R, Smith CM, Clark FJ, et al. The number of human peripheral blood CD4+ CD25high regulatory T cells increases with age. *Clin. Exp. Immunol.* Jun 2005;140(3):540-546.

[63] Trzonkowski P, Szmit E, Mysliwska J, Mysliwski A. CD4+CD25+ T regulatory cells inhibit cytotoxic activity of CTL and NK cells in humans-impact of immunosenescence. *Clin Immunol.* Jun 2006;119(3):307-316.

[64] Solana R, Pawelec G, Tarazona R. Aging and innate immunity. *Immunity.* May 2006;24(5):491-494.

[65] Ginaldi L, De Martinis M, D'Ostilio A, Marini L, Loreto MF, Quaglino D. The immune system in the elderly: III. Innate immunity. *Immunol. Res.* 1999;20(2):117-126.

[66] de la Fuente M, Hernanz A, Guayerbas N, Alvarez P, Alvarado C. Changes with age in peritoneal macrophage functions. Implication of leukocytes in the oxidative stress of senescence. *Cell Mol. Biol. (Noisy-le-grand).* 2004;50 Online Pub:OL683-690.

[67] De la Fuente M, Hernanz A, Guayerbas N, Victor VM, Arnalich F. Vitamin E ingestion improves several immune functions in elderly men and women. *Free Radic Res.* Mar 2008;42(3):272-280.

[68] Gomez CR, Nomellini V, Faunce DE, Kovacs EJ. Innate immunity and aging. *Exp. Gerontol.* Aug 2008;43(8):718-728.

[69] Lord JM, Butcher S, Killampali V, Lascelles D, Salmon M. Neutrophil ageing and immunesenescence. *Mech. Ageing Dev.* Sep 30 2001;122(14):1521-1535.

[70] Rafi A, Castle SC, Uyemura K, Makinodan T. Immune dysfunction in the elderly and its reversal by antihistamines. *Biomed Pharmacother.* Jul-Aug 2003;57(5-6):246-250.

[71] Linton PJ, Dorshkind K. Age-related changes in lymphocyte development and function. *Nat. Immunol.* Feb 2004;5(2):133-139.

[72] Castle SC, Uyemura K, Fulop T, Makinodan T. Host resistance and immune responses in advanced age. *Clin Geriatr Med.* Aug 2007;23(3):463-479, v.

[73] De La Fuente M. Changes in the macrophage function with aging. *Comp. Biochem. Physiol. A Comp. Physiol.* 1985;81(4):935-938.

[74] Ogata K, An E, Shioi Y, et al. Association between natural killer cell activity and infection in immunologically normal elderly people. *Clin. Exp. Immunol.* Jun 2001;124(3):392-397.

[75] Niwa Y, Kasama T, Miyachi Y, Kanoh T. Neutrophil chemotaxis, phagocytosis and parameters of reactive oxygen species in human aging: cross-sectional and longitudinal studies. *Life Sci.* 1989;44(22):1655-1664.

[76] van Duin D, Allore HG, Mohanty S, et al. Prevaccine determination of the expression of costimulatory B7 molecules in activated monocytes predicts influenza vaccine responses in young and older adults. *J. Infect. Dis.* Jun 1 2007;195(11):1590-1597.

[77] Kong KF, Delroux K, Wang X, et al. Dysregulation of TLR3 impairs the innate immune response to West Nile virus in the elderly. *J. Virol.* Aug 2008;82(15):7613-7623.

[78] Solana R, Alonso MC, Pena J. Natural killer cells in healthy aging. *Exp. Gerontol.* Jun 1999;34(3):435-443.

[79] Mocchegiani E, Malavolta M. NK and NKT cell functions in immunosenescence. *Aging Cell.* Aug 2004;3(4):177-184.

[80] Plackett TP, Boehmer ED, Faunce DE, Kovacs EJ. Aging and innate immune cells. *J. Leukoc. Biol.* Aug 2004;76(2):291-299.

[81] Shodell M, Siegal FP. Circulating, interferon-producing plasmacytoid dendritic cells decline during human ageing. *Scand. J. Immunol.* Nov 2002;56(5):518-521.

[82] De la Fuente M. Effects of antioxidants on immune system ageing. *Eur. J. Clin. Nutr.* Aug 2002;56 Suppl 3:S5-8.

[83] Villanueva JL, Solana R, Alonso MC, Pena J. Changes in the expression of HLA-class II antigens on peripheral blood monocytes from aged humans. *Dis Markers.* Mar-Apr 1990;8(2):85-91.

[84] Njemini R, Lambert M, Demanet C, Mets T. Heat shock protein 32 in human peripheral blood mononuclear cells: effect of aging and inflammation. *J. Clin. Immunol.* Sep 2005;25(5):405-417.

[85] Mollinedo F, Borregaard N, Boxer LA. Novel trends in neutrophil structure, function and development. *Immunol Today.* Dec 1999;20(12):535-537.

[86] Aird WC. The role of the endothelium in severe sepsis and multiple organ dysfunction syndrome. *Blood.* May 15 2003;101(10):3765-3777.

[87] van den Berg JM, Weyer S, Weening JJ, Roos D, Kuijpers TW. Divergent effects of tumor necrosis factor alpha on apoptosis of human neutrophils. *J. Leukoc. Biol.* Mar 2001;69(3):467-473.

[88] Fortin CF, McDonald PP, Lesur O, Fulop T, Jr. Aging and neutrophils: there is still much to do. *Rejuvenation Res.* Oct 2008;11(5):873-882.

[89] Schroder AK, Rink L. Neutrophil immunity of the elderly. *Mech. Ageing Dev.* Apr 2003;124(4):419-425.

[90] Fortin CF, Lesur O, Fulop T, Jr. Effects of aging on triggering receptor expressed on myeloid cells (TREM)-1-induced PMN functions. *FEBS Lett.* Mar 20 2007;581(6):1173-1178.

[91] Segal AW, Abo A. The biochemical basis of the NADPH oxidase of phagocytes. *Trends Biochem. Sci.* Feb 1993;18(2):43-47.

[92] Meydani SN, Wu D, Santos MS, Hayek MG. Antioxidants and immune response in aged persons: overview of present evidence. *Am. J. Clin. Nutr.* Dec 1995;62(6 Suppl):1462S-1476S.

[93] Carmody RJ, Cotter TG. Signalling apoptosis: a radical approach. *Redox. Rep.* 2001;6(2):77-90.

[94] Kinnula VL, Soini Y, Kvist-Makela K, Savolainen ER, Koistinen P. Antioxidant defense mechanisms in human neutrophils. *Antioxid .Redox. Signal.* Feb 2002;4(1):27-34.

[95] Roos D, Weening RS, Voetman AA. Protection of human neutrophils against oxidative damage. *Agents Actions.* Dec 1980;10(6):528-535.

[96] Narayanan PK, Ragheb K, Lawler G, Robinson JP. Defects in intracellular oxidative metabolism of neutrophils undergoing apoptosis. *J. Leukoc. Biol.* Apr 1997;61(4):481-488.

[97] O'Neill AJ, O'Neill S, Hegarty NJ, et al. Glutathione depletion-induced neutrophil apoptosis is caspase 3 dependent. *Shock.* Dec 2000;14(6):605-609.

[98] Ogino T, Packer L, Maguire JJ. Neutrophil antioxidant capacity during the respiratory burst: loss of glutathione induced by chloramines. *Free Radic. Biol. Med.* 1997;23(3):445-452.

[99] van den Dobbelsteen DJ, Nobel CS, Schlegel J, Cotgreave IA, Orrenius S, Slater AF. Rapid and specific efflux of reduced glutathione during apoptosis induced by anti-Fas/APO-1 antibody. *J. Biol. Chem.* Jun 28 1996;271(26):15420-15427.

[100] Watson RW, Rotstein OD, Jimenez M, Parodo J, Marshall JC. Augmented intracellular glutathione inhibits Fas-triggered apoptosis of activated human neutrophils. *Blood.* Jun 1 1997;89(11):4175-4181.

[101] Scheel-Toellner D, Wang K, Craddock R, et al. Reactive oxygen species limit neutrophil life span by activating death receptor signaling. *Blood.* Oct 15 2004;104(8):2557-2564.

[102] Alonso-Fernandez P, Puerto M, Mate I, Ribera JM, de la Fuente M. Neutrophils of centenarians show function levels similar to those of young adults. *J. Am. Geriatr. Soc.* Dec 2008;56(12):2244-2251.
[103] Ligthart GJ, Corberand JX, Fournier C, et al. Admission criteria for immunogerontological studies in man: the SENIEUR protocol. *Mech. Ageing Dev.* Nov 1984;28(1):47-55.
[104] Ferrandez MD, De la Fuente M. Effects of age, sex and physical exercise on the phagocytic process of murine peritoneal macrophages. *Acta Physiol. Scand.* May 1999;166(1):47-53.
[105] Esparza B, Sanchez H, Ruiz M, Barranquero M, Sabino E, Merino F. Neutrophil function in elderly persons assessed by flow cytometry. *Immunol. Invest.* May 1996;25(3):185-190.
[106] Alvarez E, Ruiz-Gutierrez V, Sobrino F, Santa-Maria C. Age-related changes in membrane lipid composition, fluidity and respiratory burst in rat peritoneal neutrophils. *Clin. Exp. Immunol.* Apr 2001;124(1):95-102.
[107] Zou Y, Jung KJ, Kim JW, Yu BP, Chung HY. Alteration of soluble adhesion molecules during aging and their modulation by calorie restriction. *FASEB J.* Feb 2004;18(2):320-322.
[108] Simons K, Toomre D. Lipid rafts and signal transduction. *Nat. Rev. Mol. Cell Biol.* Oct 2000;1(1):31-39.
[109] Fortin CF, Larbi A, Lesur O, Douziech N, Fulop T, Jr. Impairment of SHP-1 down-regulation in the lipid rafts of human neutrophils under GM-CSF stimulation contributes to their age-related, altered functions. *J. Leukoc Biol.* May 2006;79(5):1061-1072.
[110] Fulop T, Larbi A, Douziech N, et al. Signal transduction and functional changes in neutrophils with aging. *Aging Cell.* Aug 2004;3(4):217-226.
[111] Tortorella C, Simone O, Piazzolla G, Stella I, Antonaci S. Age-related impairment of GM-CSF-induced signalling in neutrophils: role of SHP-1 and SOCS proteins. *Ageing Res. Rev.* Aug 2007;6(2):81-93.
[112] Tortorella C, Simone O, Piazzolla G, Stella I, Cappiello V, Antonaci S. Role of phosphoinositide 3-kinase and extracellular signal-regulated kinase pathways in granulocyte macrophage-colony-stimulating factor failure to delay fas-induced neutrophil apoptosis in elderly humans. *J Gerontol A Biol. Sci. Med. Sci.* Nov 2006;61(11):1111-1118.
[113] Larbi A, Fulop T, Pawelec G. Immune receptor signaling, aging and autoimmunity. *Adv. Exp. Med. Biol.* 2008;640:312-324.
[114] Polignano A, Tortorella C, Venezia A, Jirillo E, Antonaci S. Age-associated changes of neutrophil responsiveness in a human healthy elderly population. *Cytobios.* 1994;80(322):145-153.

[115] Wenisch C, Patruta S, Daxbock F, Krause R, Horl W. Effect of age on human neutrophil function. *J. Leukoc. Biol.* Jan 2000;67(1):40-45.

[116] Egger G, Aigner R, Glasner A, Hofer HP, Mitterhammer H, Zelzer S. Blood polymorphonuclear leukocyte migration as a predictive marker for infections in severe trauma: comparison with various inflammation parameters. *Intensive Care Med.* Feb 2004;30(2):331-334.

[117] Egger G, Burda A, Mitterhammer H, Baumann G, Bratschitsch G, Glasner A. Impaired blood polymorphonuclear leukocyte migration and infection risk in severe trauma. *J. Infect.* Aug 2003;47(2):148-154.

[118] Viveros MP, Arranz L, Hernanz A, Miquel J, De la Fuente M. A model of premature aging in mice based on altered stress-related behavioral response and immunosenescence. *Neuroimmunomodulation.* 2007;14(3-4):157-162.

[119] Butcher SK, Chahal H, Nayak L, et al. Senescence in innate immune responses: reduced neutrophil phagocytic capacity and CD16 expression in elderly humans. *J. Leukoc. Biol.* Dec 2001;70(6):881-886.

[120] Suzuki M, Miura S, Mori M, et al. Rebamipide, a novel antiulcer agent, attenuates Helicobacter pylori induced gastric mucosal cell injury associated with neutrophil derived oxidants. *Gut.* Oct 1994;35(10):1375-1378.

[121] Arranz L, Fernandez C, Rodriguez A, Ribera JM, De la Fuente M. The glutathione precursor N-acetylcysteine improves immune function in postmenopausal women. *Free Radic. Biol .Med.* Nov 1 2008;45(9):1252-1262.

[122] Sohal RS, Farmer KJ, Allen RG. Correlates of longevity in two strains of the housefly, Musca domestica. *Mech. Ageing. Dev.* Sep 30 1987;40(2):171-179.

[123] Sohal RS, Ku HH, Agarwal S. Biochemical correlates of longevity in two closely related rodent species. *Biochem. Biophys. Res. Commun.* Oct 15 1993;196(1):7-11.

[124] Fulop T, Jr., Varga Z, Jacob MP, Robert L. Effect of lithium on superoxide production and intracellular free calcium mobilization in elastin peptide (kappa-elastin) and FMLP stimulated human PMNS. Effect of age. *Life Sci.* 1997;60(22):PL 325-332.

[125] Rao KM. Age-related decline in ligand-induced actin polymerization in human leukocytes and platelets. *J. Gerontol.* Sep 1986;41(5):561-566.

[126] Piazzolla G, Tortorella C, Serrone M, Jirillo E, Antonaci S. Modulation of cytoskeleton assembly capacity and oxidative response in aged

neutrophils. *Immunopharmaco.l Immunotoxicol.* May 1998;20(2):251-266.

[127] Radsak MP, Salih HR, Rammensee HG, Schild H. Triggering receptor expressed on myeloid cells-1 in neutrophil inflammatory responses: differential regulation of activation and survival. *J. Immunol.* Apr 15 2004;172(8):4956-4963.

[128] Pawelec G. Immunity and ageing in man. *Exp. Gerontol.* Dec 2006;41(12):1239-1242.

[129] Puerto M, Guayerbas N, Alvarez P, De la Fuente M. Modulation of neuropeptide Y and norepinephrine on several leucocyte functions in adult, old and very old mice. *J. Neuroimmunol.* Aug 2005;165(1-2):33-40.

[130] Kalpakcioglu B, Senel K. The interrelation of glutathione reductase, catalase, glutathione peroxidase, superoxide dismutase, and glucose-6-phosphate in the pathogenesis of rheumatoid arthritis. *Clin. Rheumatol.* Feb 2008;27(2):141-145.

[131] Gambhir JK, Lali P, Jain AK. Correlation between blood antioxidant levels and lipid peroxidation in rheumatoid arthritis. *Clin. Biochem.* Jun 1997;30(4):351-355.

[132] Droge W, Pottmeyer-Gerber C, Schmidt H, Nick S. Glutathione augments the activation of cytotoxic T lymphocytes in vivo. *Immunobiology.* Aug 1986;172(1-2):151-156.

[133] Staal FJ, Roederer M, Herzenberg LA. Intracellular thiols regulate activation of nuclear factor kappa B and transcription of human immunodeficiency virus. *Proc. Natl. Acad. Sci. U S A.* Dec 1990;87(24):9943-9947.

[134] Mihm S, Galter D, Droge W. Modulation of transcription factor NF kappa B activity by intracellular glutathione levels and by variations of the extracellular cysteine supply. *FASEB J.* Feb 1995;9(2):246-252.

[135] Tewes F, Bol GF, Brigelius-Flohe R. Thiol modulation inhibits the interleukin (IL)-1-mediated activation of an IL-1 receptor-associated protein kinase and NF-kappa B. *Eur. J. Immunol.* Nov 1997;27(11):3015-3021.

[136] Collard CD, Vakeva A, Bukusoglu C, et al. Reoxygenation of hypoxic human umbilical vein endothelial cells activates the classic complement pathway. *Circulation.* Jul 1 1997;96(1):326-333.

[137] Collard CD, Agah A, Stahl GL. Complement activation following reoxygenation of hypoxic human endothelial cells: role of intracellular

reactive oxygen species, NF-kappaB and new protein synthesis. *Immunopharmacology.* Mar 1998;39(1):39-50.

[138] Pastore A, Federici G, Bertini E, Piemonte F. Analysis of glutathione: implication in redox and detoxification. *Clin. Chim. Acta.* Jul 1 2003;333(1):19-39.

[139] Burek CL, Rose NR. Autoimmune thyroiditis and ROS. *Autoimmun. Rev.* Jul 2008;7(7):530-537.

[140] Lang CA, Mills BJ, Lang HL, et al. High blood glutathione levels accompany excellent physical and mental health in women ages 60 to 103 years. *J. Lab Clin. Med.* Dec 2002;140(6):413-417.

[141] Bhushan M, Cumberbatch M, Dearman RJ, Andrew SM, Kimber I, Griffiths CE. Tumour necrosis factor-alpha-induced migration of human Langerhans cells: the influence of ageing. *Br. J. Dermatol.* Jan 2002;146(1):32-40.

[142] Droge W, Kinscherf R. Aberrant insulin receptor signaling and amino acid homeostasis as a major cause of oxidative stress in aging. *Antioxid. Redox. Signal.* Apr 2008;10(4):661-678.

[143] Kulinsky VI. Biochemical aspects of inflammation. *Biochemistry (Mosc).* Jun 2007;72(6):595-607.

[144] Csiszar A, Wang M, Lakatta EG, Ungvari Z. Inflammation and endothelial dysfunction during aging: role of NF-kappaB. *J. Appl. Physiol.* Oct 2008;105(4):1333-1341.

[145] Libby P. Inflammatory mechanisms: the molecular basis of inflammation and disease. *Nutr. Rev.* Dec 2007;65(12 Pt 2):S140-146.

[146] Yuan H, Zheng JC, Liu P, Zhang SF, Xu JY, Bai LM. Pathogenesis of Parkinson's disease: oxidative stress, environmental impact factors and inflammatory processes. *Neurosci Bull.* Mar 2007;23(2):125-130.

[147] Chung HY, Sung B, Jung KJ, Zou Y, Yu BP. The molecular inflammatory process in aging. *Antioxid Redox Signal.* Mar-Apr 2006;8(3-4):572-581.

[148] Franceschi C. Inflammaging as a major characteristic of old people: can it be prevented or cured? *Nutr. Rev.* Dec 2007;65(12 Pt 2):S173-176.

[149] Ostan R, Bucci L, Capri M, et al. Immunosenescence and immunogenetics of human longevity. *Neuroimmunomodulation.* 2008;15(4-6):224-240.

[150] Meydani SN, Wu D. Age-associated inflammatory changes: role of nutritional intervention. *Nutr. Rev.* Dec 2007;65(12 Pt 2):S213-216.

[151] Barnes PJ, Karin M. Nuclear factor-kappaB: a pivotal transcription factor in chronic inflammatory diseases. *N. Engl. J. Med.* Apr 10 1997;336(15):1066-1071.

[152] Victor VM, De la Fuente M. Immune cells redox state from mice with endotoxin-induced oxidative stress. Involvement of NF-kappaB. *Free Radic Res.* Jan 2003;37(1):19-27.

[153] Victor VM, Rocha M, Esplugues JV, De la Fuente M. Role of free radicals in sepsis: antioxidant therapy. *Curr. Pharm. Des.* 2005;11(24):3141-3158.

[154] Gwinn MR, Vallyathan V. Respiratory burst: role in signal transduction in alveolar macrophages. *J. Toxicol. Environ. Health B Crit Rev.* Jan-Feb 2006;9(1):27-39.

[155] Trebilcock GU, Ponnappan U. Evidence for lowered induction of nuclear factor kappa B in activated human T lymphocytes during aging. *Gerontology.* 1996;42(3):137-146.

[156] Salminen A, Huuskonen J, Ojala J, Kauppinen A, Kaarniranta K, Suuronen T. Activation of innate immunity system during aging: NF-kB signaling is the molecular culprit of inflamm-aging. *Ageing Res. Rev.* Apr 2008;7(2):83-105.

[157] Salminen A, Kauppinen A, Suuronen T, Kaarniranta K. SIRT1 longevity factor suppresses NF-kappaB -driven immune responses: regulation of aging via NF-kappaB acetylation? *Bioessays.* Oct 2008;30(10):939-942.

[158] De Martinis M, Franceschi C, Monti D, Ginaldi L. Inflammation markers predicting frailty and mortality in the elderly. *Exp. Mol. Pathol.* Jun 2006;80(3):219-227.

[159] De Martinis M, Franceschi C, Monti D, Ginaldi L. Inflamm-ageing and lifelong antigenic load as major determinants of ageing rate and longevity. *FEBS Lett.* Apr 11 2005;579(10):2035-2039.

[160] Ferencik M, Stvrtinova V, Hulin I, Novak M. Inflammation--a lifelong companion. Attempt at a non-analytical holistic view. *Folia Microbiol (Praha).* 2007;52(2):159-173.

[161] Paolisso G, Barbieri M, Bonafe M, Franceschi C. Metabolic age modelling: the lesson from centenarians. *Eur. J. Clin. Invest.* Oct 2000;30(10):888-894.

[162] Franceschi C, Monti D, Sansoni P, Cossarizza A. The immunology of exceptional individuals: the lesson of centenarians. *Immunol. Today.* Jan 1995;16(1):12-16.

[163] Miyaji C, Watanabe H, Toma H, et al. Functional alteration of granulocytes, NK cells, and natural killer T cells in centenarians. *Hum. Immunol.* Sep 2000;61(9):908-916.

[164] Schriner SE, Linford NJ, Martin GM, et al. Extension of murine life span by overexpression of catalase targeted to mitochondria. *Science.* Jun 24 2005;308(5730):1909-1911.

[165] Balbis E, Patriarca S, Furfaro AL, et al. Oxidative stress and antioxidant defence in a healthy nonagenarian population. *Redox. Rep.* 2007;12(1):59-62.

[166] De la Fuente M, Baeza I, Guayerbas N, et al. Changes with ageing in several leukocyte functions of male and female rats. *Biogerontology.* 2004;5(6):389-400.

[167] Vina J, Sastre J, Pallardo FV, Gambini J, Borras C. Role of mitochondrial oxidative stress to explain the different longevity between genders: protective effect of estrogens. *Free Radic. Res.* Dec 2006;40(12):1359-1365.

[168] Ali SS, Xiong C, Lucero J, Behrens MM, Dugan LL, Quick KL. Gender differences in free radical homeostasis during aging: shorter-lived female C57BL6 mice have increased oxidative stress. *Aging Cell.* Dec 2006;5(6):565-574.

[169] Borras C, Gambini J, Vina J. Mitochondrial oxidant generation is involved in determining why females live longer than males. *Front Biosci.* 2007;12:1008-1013.

[170] Giraldo E, Hinchado MD, Garcia JJ, Ortega E. Influence of gender and oral contraceptives intake on innate and inflammatory response. Role of neuroendocrine factors. *Mol. Cell Biochem.* Jun 2008;313(1-2):147-153.

[171] Vasto S, Candore G, Balistreri CR, et al. Inflammatory networks in ageing, age-related diseases and longevity. *Mech. Ageing Dev.* Jan 2007;128(1):83-91.

[172] Haus E, Lakatua DJ, Swoyer J, Sackett-Lundeen L. Chronobiology in hematology and immunology. *Am J Anat.* Dec 1983;168(4):467-517.

[173] Haus E. Chronobiology in the endocrine system. *Adv. Drug Deliv. Rev.* Aug 31 2007;59(9-10):985-1014.

[174] Esquifino AI, Cano P, Jimenez-Ortega V, Fernandez-Mateos P, Cardinali DP. Neuroendocrine-immune correlates of circadian physiology: studies in experimental models of arthritis, ethanol feeding, aging, social isolation, and calorie restriction. *Endocrine.* Aug 2007;32(1):1-19.

[175] Rodriguez AB, Marchena JM, Nogales G, Duran J, Barriga C. Correlation between the circadian rhythm of melatonin, phagocytosis, and superoxide anion levels in ring dove heterophils. *J. Pineal. Res.* Jan 1999;26(1):35-42.

[176] Terron MP, Paredes SD, Barriga C, Ortega E, Rodriguez AB. Comparative study of the heterophil phagocytic function in young and old ring doves (Streptopelia risoria) and its relationship with melatonin levels. *J. Comp. Physiol. B.* Jul 2004;174(5):421-427.

[177] Cardinali DP, Garcia AP, Cano P, Esquifino AI. Melatonin role in experimental arthritis. *Curr Drug Targets Immune Endocr. Metabol. Disord.* Mar 2004;4(1):1-10.

[178] Srinivasan V, Spence DW, Trakht I, Pandi-Perumal SR, Cardinali DP, Maestroni GJ. Immunomodulation by melatonin: its significance for seasonally occurring diseases. *Neuroimmunomodulation.* 2008;15(2):93-101.

[179] De la Fuente M. and Diaz B. *Melatonin, aging and health.* New York: Nova Science Publishers, Inc.; 2007.

[180] Paredes SD, Terron MP, Marchena AM, et al. Effect of exogenous melatonin on viability, ingestion capacity, and free-radical scavenging in heterophils from young and old ringdoves (Streptopelia risoria). *Mol Cell Biochem.* Oct 2007;304(1-2):305-314.

[181] Cardinali DP, Esquifino AI, Srinivasan V, Pandi-Perumal SR. Melatonin and the immune system in aging. *Neuroimmunomodulation.* 2008;15(4-6):272-278.

[182] Grubeck-Loebenstein B, Berger P, Saurwein-Teissl M, Zisterer K, Wick G. No immunity for the elderly. *Nat. Med.* Aug 1998;4(8):870.

[183] Castle SC. Clinical relevance of age-related immune dysfunction. *Clin. Infect. Dis.* Aug 2000;31(2):578-585.

[184] El Yousfi M, Mercier S, Breuille D, et al. The inflammatory response to vaccination is altered in the elderly. *Mech. Ageing Dev.* Aug 2005;126(8):874-881.

[185] McElhaney JE. Overcoming the challenges of immunosenescence in the prevention of acute respiratory illness in older people. *Conn. Med.* Sep 2003;67(8):469-474.

[186] Hasler P, Zouali M. Immune receptor signaling, aging, and autoimmunity. *Cell Immunol.* Feb 2005;233(2):102-108.

[187] Licastro F, Candore G, Lio D, et al. Innate immunity and inflammation in ageing: a key for understanding age-related diseases. *Immun. Ageing.* May 18 2005;2:8.

[188] McGeer PL, McGeer EG. Inflammation and the degenerative diseases of aging. *Ann. N Y Acad. Sci.* Dec 2004;1035:104-116.

[189] McGeer EG, Klegeris A, McGeer PL. Inflammation, the complement system and the diseases of aging. *Neurobiol Aging.* Dec 2005;26 Suppl 1:94-97.

[190] Franceschi C, Bonafe M, Valensin S, et al. Inflamm-aging. An evolutionary perspective on immunosenescence. *Ann. N Y Acad. Sci.* Jun 2000;908:244-254.

[191] Wick G, Jansen-Durr P, Berger P, Blasko I, Grubeck-Loebenstein B. Diseases of aging. *Vaccine.* Feb 25 2000;18(16):1567-1583.

[192] Ben-Yehuda A, Weksler ME. Immune senescence: mechanisms and clinical implications. *Cancer Invest.* 1992;10(6):525-531.

[193] Sarkar D, Fisher PB. Molecular mechanisms of aging-associated inflammation. *Cancer Lett.* May 8 2006;236(1):13-23.

[194] Paulus WJ. Cytokines and heart failure. *Heart Fail Monit.* 2000;1(2):50-56.

[195] Mangge H, Hubmann H, Pilz S, Schauenstein K, Renner W, Marz W. Beyond cholesterol--inflammatory cytokines, the key mediators in atherosclerosis. *Clin. Chem. Lab. Med.* May 2004;42(5):467-474.

[196] Wisse BE. The inflammatory syndrome: the role of adipose tissue cytokines in metabolic disorders linked to obesity. *J Am Soc Nephrol.* Nov 2004;15(11):2792-2800.

[197] Aukrust P, Gullestad L, Ueland T, Damas JK, Yndestad A. Inflammatory and anti-inflammatory cytokines in chronic heart failure: potential therapeutic implications. *Ann. Med.* 2005;37(2):74-85.

[198] van Baarle D, Tsegaye A, Miedema F, Akbar A. Significance of senescence for virus-specific memory T cell responses: rapid ageing during chronic stimulation of the immune system. *Immunol Lett.* Feb 15 2005;97(1):19-29.

[199] Koch S, Solana R, Dela Rosa O, Pawelec G. Human cytomegalovirus infection and T cell immunosenescence: a mini review. *Mech. Ageing Dev.* Jun 2006;127(6):538-543.

[200] Franceschi C, Capri M, Monti D, et al. Inflammaging and anti-inflammaging: a systemic perspective on aging and longevity emerged from studies in humans. *Mech. Ageing Dev.* Jan 2007;128(1):92-105.

[201] Van Bodegom D, May L, Meij HJ, Westendorp RG. Regulation of human life histories: the role of the inflammatory host response. *Ann N Y Acad Sci.* Apr 2007;1100:84-97.

[202] Vasto S, Carruba G, Lio D, et al. Inflammation, ageing and cancer. *Mech Ageing Dev.* Jan-Feb 2009;130(1-2):40-45.

[203] Ottaviani E, Malagoli D, Capri M, Franceschi C. Ecoimmunology: is there any room for the neuroendocrine system? *Bioessays.* Sep 2008;30(9):868-874.

[204] Finch CE, Crimmins EM. Inflammatory exposure and historical changes in human life-spans. *Science.* Sep 17 2004;305(5691):1736-1739.

[205] Crimmins EM, Finch CE. Infection, inflammation, height, and longevity. *Proc. Natl. Acad. Sci. U S A.* Jan 10 2006;103(2):498-503.

[206] Miquel J. Can antioxidant diet supplementation protect against age-related mitochondrial damage? *Ann N Y Acad Sci.* Apr 2002;959:508-516.

[207] Forsberg L, de Faire U, Morgenstern R. Oxidative stress, human genetic variation, and disease. *Arch. Biochem. Biophys.* May 1 2001;389(1):84-93.

[208] Guayerbas N, Puerto M, Hernanz A, Miquel J, De la Fuente M. Thiolic antioxidant supplementation of the diet reverses age-related behavioural dysfunction in prematurely ageing mice. *Pharmacol. Biochem. Behav.* Jan 2005;80(1):45-51.

[209] De la Fuente M, Ferrandez MD, Burgos MS, Soler A, Prieto A, Miquel J. Immune function in aged women is improved by ingestion of vitamins C and E. *Can. J. Physiol Pharmacol.* Apr 1998;76(4):373-380.

[210] Puerto M, Guayerbas N, Victor V, De la Fuente M. Effects of N-acetylcysteine on macrophage and lymphocyte functions in a mouse model of premature ageing. *Pharmacol Biochem. Behav.* Nov 2002;73(4):797-804.

[211] de la Fuente M, Ferrandez D, Munoz F, de Juan E, Miquel J. Stimulation by the antioxidant thioproline of the lymphocyte functions of old mice. *Mech Ageing Dev.* May 1993;68(1-3):27-36.

[212] De la Fuente M, Ferrandez MD, Del Rio M, Sol Burgos M, Miquel J. Enhancement of leukocyte functions in aged mice supplemented with the antioxidant thioproline. *Mech. Ageing Dev.* Sep 1 1998;104(3):213-225.

[213] Correa R, Blanco B, Del Rio M, et al. Effect of a diet supplemented with thioproline on murine macrophage function in a model of premature ageing. *Biofactors.* 1999;10(2-3):195-200.

[214] De La Fuente M, Miquel J, Catalan MP, Victor VM, Guayerbas N. The amount of thiolic antioxidant ingestion needed to improve several

immune functions is higher in aged than in adult mice. *Free Radic. Res.* Feb 2002;36(2):119-126.

[215] Guayerbas N, Puerto M, Ferrandez MD, De La Fuente M. A diet supplemented with thiolic anti-oxidants improves leucocyte function in two strains of prematurely ageing mice. *Clin. Exp. Pharmacol. Physiol.* Nov 2002;29(11):1009-1014.

[216] Guayerbas N, Puerto M, Alvarez P, de la Fuente M. Improvement of the macrophage functions in prematurely ageing mice by a diet supplemented with thiolic antioxidants. *Cell Mol Biol (Noisy-le-grand).* 2004;50 Online Pub:OL677-681.

[217] Alvarado C, Alvarez P, Jimenez L, De la Fuente M. Improvement of leukocyte functions in young prematurely aging mice after a 5-week ingestion of a diet supplemented with biscuits enriched in antioxidants. *Antioxid Redox Signal.* Sep-Oct 2005;7(9-10):1203-1210.

[218] Alvarez P, Alvarado C, Puerto M, Schlumberger A, Jimenez L, De la Fuente M. Improvement of leukocyte functions in prematurely aging mice after five weeks of diet supplementation with polyphenol-rich cereals. *Nutrition.* Sep 2006;22(9):913-921.

[219] Alvarado C, Alvarez P, Puerto M, Gausseres N, Jimenez L, De la Fuente M. Dietary supplementation with antioxidants improves functions and decreases oxidative stress of leukocytes from prematurely aging mice. *Nutrition.* Jul-Aug 2006;22(7-8):767-777.

[220] Baeza I, de Castro NM, Alvarado C, et al. Improvement of immune cell functions in aged mice treated for five weeks with soybean isoflavones. *Ann. N Y Acad. Sci.* Apr 2007;1100:497-504.

[221] Hernanz A, Collazos ME, de la Fuente M. Effect of age, culture medium and lymphocyte presence on ascorbate content of peritoneal macrophages from mice and guinea pigs during phagocytosis. *Int Arch Allergy Appl. Immunol.* 1990;91(2):166-170.

[222] Blanco B, Ferrandez MD, Correa R, et al. Changes in several functions of murine peritoneal macrophages by N-acetylcysteine and thioproline ingestion. Comparative effect between two strains of mice. *Biofactors.* 1999;10(2-3):179-185.

[223] De la Fuente M, Carazo M, Correa R, Del Rio M. Changes in macrophage and lymphocyte functions in guinea-pigs after different amounts of vitamin E ingestion. *Br. J. Nutr.* Jul 2000;84(1):25-29.

[224] Alvarez P, Alvarado C, Mathieu F, Jimenez L, De la Fuente M. Diet supplementation for 5 weeks with polyphenol-rich cereals improves

several functions and the redox state of mouse leucocytes. *Eur. J. Nutr.* Dec 2006;45(8):428-438.

[225] De la Fuente M, Victor VM. Anti-oxidants as modulators of immune function. *Immunol. Cell Biol.* Feb 2000;78(1):49-54.

[226] Sastre J, Pallardo FV, Garcia de la Asuncion J, Vina J. Mitochondria, oxidative stress and aging. *Free Radic Res.* Mar 2000;32(3):189-198.

[227] Polidori MC, Mecocci P, Cherubini A, Senin U. Physical activity and oxidative stress during aging. *Int. J. Sports Med.* Apr 2000;21(3):154-157.

[228] Pedersen BK, Hoffman-Goetz L. Exercise and the immune system: regulation, integration, and adaptation. *Physiol. Rev.* Jul 2000;80(3):1055-1081.

[229] Ortega E, Collazos ME, Barriga C, De la Fuente M. Stimulation of the phagocytic function in guinea pig peritoneal macrophages by physical activity stress. *Eur. J. Appl. Physiol. Occup. Physiol.* 1992;64(4):323-327.

[230] Giraldo E, Garcia JJ, Hinchado MD, Ortega E. Exercise intensity-dependent changes in the inflammatory response in sedentary women: role of neuroendocrine parameters in the neutrophil phagocytic process and the pro-/anti-inflammatory cytokine balance. *Neuroimmunomodulation.* 2009;16(4):237-244.

[231] Ortega E. Neuroendocrine mediators in the modulation of phagocytosis by exercise: physiological implications. *Exerc. Immunol. Rev.* 2003;9:70-93.

[232] Ortega E, Giraldo E, Hinchado MD, Martin L, Garcia JJ, De la Fuente M. Neuroimmunomodulation during exercise: role of catecholamines as 'stress mediator' and/or 'danger signal' for the innate immune response. *Neuroimmunomodulation.* 2007;14(3-4):206-212.

[233] Powers SK, Ji LL, Leeuwenburgh C. Exercise training-induced alterations in skeletal muscle antioxidant capacity: a brief review. *Med. Sci. Sports Exerc.* Jul 1999;31(7):987-997.

[234] Niess AM, Dickhuth HH, Northoff H, Fehrenbach E. Free radicals and oxidative stress in exercise--immunological aspects. *Exerc. Immunol. Rev.* 1999;5:22-56.

[235] Johnson P. Antioxidant enzyme expression in health and disease: effects of exercise and hypertension. *Comp. Biochem. Physiol. C. Toxicol. Pharmacol.* Dec 2002;133(4):493-505.

[236] De la Fuente M, Hernanz A, Collazos ME, Barriga C, Ortega E. Effects of physical exercise and aging on ascorbic acid and superoxide anion

levels in peritoneal macrophages from mice and guinea pigs. *J. Comp. Physiol. B.* 1995;165(4):315-319.

[237] Smith JA, Pyne DB. Exercise, training, and neutrophil function. *Exerc. Immunol Rev.* 1997;3:96-116.

[238] Colbert LH, Visser M, Simonsick EM, et al. Physical activity, exercise, and inflammatory markers in older adults: findings from the Health, Aging and Body Composition Study. *J. Am. Geriatr. Soc.* Jul 2004;52(7):1098-1104.

[239] Arranz L, De Castro, N.M., Zambrana, C., Baeza, I., Viveros, M.P., De la Fuente, M. Improvement of leukocyte functions and redox state in ageing mice by an enriched environment. *Neuroimmunomodulation.* 2006;13:224.

Reviewed by dr. Miquel. Universidad de alicante (spain)

Index

A

acid, 24, 31, 51, 69
adaptation, 1, 38, 53, 76
adaptations, 44
adhesion, 23, 32, 43, 66
adipose, 73
adipose tissue, 73
adulthood, 37, 59
aetiology, 48
ageing population, 62
aging population, 48
aging process, 5, 6, 9, 10, 33, 38, 55, 57
agonist, 24
AIDS, 32
alcoholic liver disease, 32
alveolar macrophage, 70
amyotrophic lateral sclerosis, 32
antibody, 65
antigen, 18, 19, 27
antihistamines, 63
antioxidant, vii, 22, 25, 31, 33, 37, 39, 40, 41, 44, 49, 50, 51, 52, 53, 54, 65, 68, 70, 71, 74, 76
anxiety, 3, 15, 28
apoptosis, 21, 22, 64, 65, 66
arthritis, 71, 72
ascorbic acid, 76
assessment, 45, 59
atherosclerosis, 47, 48, 73
autoimmune diseases, vii, 15
autoimmunity, 66, 72

B

bacteria, 13
barriers, 13, 14
batteries, 27
beneficial effect, 50, 52
biological rhythms, 43
biomarkers, 6, 27, 58
brain, 28, 62
Butcher, 63, 67

C

Ca^{2+}, 26
calcium, 67
calorie, 66, 71
cancer, vii, 1, 15, 17, 47, 74
candida, 42
candida albicans, 42
cardiovascular disease, 48
carotene, 51
cataract, 32
catecholamines, 53, 76
CD8+, 27
cell line, 23

cell lines, 23
cell signaling, 24
cellular homeostasis, 37, 51
central nervous system, 62
chemokines, 21
chemotaxis, 21, 23, 25, 27, 39, 42, 44, 54, 64
cholesterol, 23, 73
chronic diseases, 32
circadian rhythm, 43, 72
circadian rhythms, 43
circulation, 19, 43
class, 19, 64
cleavage, 32
cognition, 15
collateral, 25
collateral damage, 25
complement, 13, 21, 32, 68, 73
complexity, 9, 13
composition, 24, 66
compounds, vii, 32, 33, 34, 37, 38, 50, 51, 54
consumption, 53
contraceptives, 71
cost, 6, 28
counterbalance, 38
cues, 43
culture, 75
cycles, 44
cytokines, 13, 14, 20, 21, 27, 32, 43, 47, 55, 62, 73
cytomegalovirus, 73
cytometry, 66
cytoskeleton, 67
cytotoxicity, 19

D

danger, 53, 76
death rate, 17
defects, 24
defence, 71

defense mechanisms, 65
deficiency, 32
dementia, 48
dendritic cell, 13, 18, 64
deposition, 32
depression, 15, 52
derivatives, 31
destruction, 22, 27
detoxification, 69
developed countries, 6, 37, 48
developing countries, 48
diabetes, 47
diet, 49, 50, 51, 54, 58, 74, 75
digestion, 25, 54
direct action, 44
DNA, vii, 23, 33, 61
donors, 24, 26
down-regulation, 66

E

elastin, 67
elderly population, 59, 66
endocrine, 2, 3, 15, 34, 62, 71
endocrine system, 2, 71
endocrinology, 62
endothelial cells, 68
endothelial dysfunction, 69
endothelium, 21, 23, 24, 32, 64
endotoxemia, 49
environmental conditions, 5
environmental factors, 3, 6
environmental impact, 69
environmental influences, 60
enzymes, vii, 22, 23, 32, 53
Epstein-Barr virus, 47
ester, 24
estrogen, 41
ethanol, 71
exclusion, 24
execution, 22
exercise, 52, 53, 54, 60, 76, 77

exploration, 28
exposure, 2, 74
extracellular matrix, 22

F

fragments, 32
free radicals, 22, 27, 51, 70
frequencies, 43
functional changes, 66
fungi, 13

G

gastric mucosa, 67
gender differences, viii, 41
gene expression, 19
genes, 3, 9, 10, 33, 34, 49
genetic factors, 3
genotype, 6
gerontology, 9
gland, 44
glucose, 68
glutathione, vii, 23, 31, 32, 33, 39, 50, 65, 67, 68, 69
GM-CSF, 21, 24, 66

H

half-life, 21
haplotypes, 43
happiness, 62
hazards, 6
health care costs, 1
health status, 1, 43
heart disease, 47
heart failure, 73
heat shock protein, 19
height, 74
hematology, 71
heredity, 61
high blood pressure, 47

HLA, 64
homeostasis, vii, 1, 2, 3, 5, 13, 14, 15, 34, 37, 50, 51, 57, 69, 71
host, 73
human immunodeficiency virus, 68
human leukocyte antigen, 43
human neutrophils, 24, 64, 65, 66
human subjects, 17, 28, 29, 38, 49, 50
humoral immunity, 17, 44
hydrogen, 25
hydrogen peroxide, 25
hypertension, 61, 76
hypothesis, 15

I

IFN, 19
immune function, viii, 1, 2, 7, 14, 17, 18, 27, 28, 33, 35, 41, 44, 50, 52, 53, 58, 62, 63, 67, 75, 76
immune response, 2, 14, 18, 19, 33, 38, 44, 47, 52, 53, 62, 63, 64, 65, 67, 70, 76
immunity, 2, 13, 14, 18, 19, 23, 38, 47, 55, 60, 63, 65, 72
immunogenetics, 69
immunomodulatory, 44
immunosuppression, 52
impacts, 47
impairments, 1
in vivo, 68
incidence, 1, 47, 59
induction, 22, 70
inflammation, 21, 22, 25, 31, 32, 33, 34, 35, 37, 47, 48, 50, 54, 61, 64, 67, 69, 72, 73, 74
inflammatory cells, 22
inflammatory disease, 33, 48, 70
inflammatory mediators, 22, 48
inflammatory responses, 14, 68
influenza vaccine, 64
ingestion, 25, 27, 49, 50, 54, 63, 72, 74, 75
inhibition, 24, 31

initiation, 18, 23
innate immunity, 2, 14, 18, 38, 63, 70
insulin, 69
integration, 76
interferon, 64
intervention, 21, 55, 69
invertebrates, 38
isolation, 50, 71

K

killer cells, 60, 64

L

Langerhans cells, 69
leucocyte, 68, 75
life expectancy, vii, 1, 6, 34, 41, 48
ligand, 67
lipid peroxidation, 68
lipids, 23, 33
lithium, 67
longitudinal study, 6, 60
lymphocytes, 14, 18, 27, 33, 38, 55, 62
lymphoid, 14
lymphoid tissue, 14

M

macromolecules, 22
macrophages, 3, 13, 18, 19, 22, 23, 25, 38, 42, 50, 54, 62, 66, 75, 76, 77
macular degeneration, 47
majority, 7
markers, viii, 2, 3, 27, 28, 40, 55, 57, 70, 77
medical care, 48
melatonin, 44, 45, 72
membranes, 22
memory, 2, 14, 18, 73
mental activity, 55
mental health, 32, 39, 69
messengers, 14

metabolic disorder, 73
metabolism, 10, 31, 43, 65
MHC, 19
mice, 2, 3, 23, 25, 26, 28, 29, 33, 34, 35, 38, 39, 41, 42, 50, 51, 52, 53, 54, 55, 58, 61, 67, 68, 70, 71, 74, 75, 77
migration, 24, 67, 69
mitochondria, 10, 41, 51, 61, 71
mitochondrial damage, 74
modelling, 70
molecular oxygen, 53
molecules, 13, 14, 22, 32, 43, 60, 64, 66
morbidity, 1, 3, 15, 17, 25, 34, 47, 48, 60, 62
morphology, 10
muscular dystrophy, 32
mutation, 61
myeloid cells, 65, 68

N

natural killer cell, 13, 64
natural selection, 61
necrosis, 21, 69
negative feedback, 22
nervous system, 14, 15, 50, 51
neurodegenerative diseases, 47
neuroendocrine system, 15, 74
neurotransmitter, 14
neutrophils, vii, 3, 13, 21, 22, 23, 24, 25, 26, 31, 32, 33, 38, 39, 40, 42, 44, 45, 50, 55, 57, 65, 66, 68
Nile, 64
nitrogen, 14
NK cells, 14, 18, 19, 27, 63, 71
norepinephrine, 68
nutrition, 23

O

obesity, 73
old age, 34, 43, 48
organ, 44, 62, 64

Index

organism, vii, 1, 5, 6, 10, 13, 15, 28, 32, 34, 37, 38, 50, 51, 57
oscillations, 43
oxidation, vii, 10, 23, 31, 33, 34, 37, 42, 50, 54, 61
oxidative damage, 22, 33, 34, 53, 65
oxidative stress, viii, 3, 10, 23, 24, 32, 34, 35, 37, 39, 40, 49, 50, 52, 53, 57, 61, 63, 69, 70, 71, 75, 76
oxygen, 11, 14, 22, 32, 38, 50, 65, 69

prognosis, 45
programming, 34
pro-inflammatory, vii, 19, 21, 32, 33, 37, 38, 43, 47, 48, 55
project, 27
prostaglandins, 32
proteases, 22, 25
protein kinase C, 24, 26
protein synthesis, 69
proteins, 19, 22, 66

P

pathogenesis, 31, 32, 68
pathogens, 14, 19, 21, 27, 47, 51
pathways, 22, 31, 66
periodicity, 43
peripheral blood, vii, 19, 21, 23, 28, 33, 38, 39, 40, 55, 63, 64
peripheral blood mononuclear cell, 64
peroxide, 25
phagocytosis, 21, 23, 25, 26, 27, 42, 44, 54, 64, 72, 75, 76
phenotype, 19
phenylalanine, 21
phospholipids, 24
phosphorylation, 26
physical activity, 52, 55, 76
physical exercise, 52, 53, 54, 58, 61, 66, 76
physiology, 10, 62, 71
pineal gland, 44
plasma membrane, 23
platelets, 67
pneumonia, 1, 59
polymerization, 26, 67
polyphenols, 50
polyunsaturated fat, 22
postmenopausal women, 67
premature death, 28
prevention, 72
priming, 24
probability, 37

Q

quality of life, 52, 55

R

radiation, 61
radicals, 22, 76
reaction time, 7
reactive oxygen, 26, 37, 39, 51, 64, 69
reception, 15
receptors, 14, 19, 20, 24, 43
recognition, 14, 27
recommendations, iv
relevance, 72
REM, 65
remodelling, 59
replacement, 5
reproduction, 10, 11, 37
reproductive age, 11
reserves, 50
resistance, 14, 15, 17, 53, 63
respiration, 53
respiratory distress syndrome, 32
responsiveness, 63, 66
rheumatoid arthritis, 32, 47, 68
rhythm, 43
risk factors, 45

S

saturated fat, 24
secretion, 27, 44
selenium, 51
senescence, 9, 15, 28, 32, 38, 61, 63, 73
sepsis, 21, 64, 70
serum, 20, 44, 47, 48
sex, 28, 43, 66
sexual reproduction, 5, 11
shock, 64
signal transduction, 66, 70
signaling pathway, 19, 24
signalling, 66
signals, 19, 53
skeletal muscle, 53, 76
species, 5, 6, 9, 11, 14, 22, 26, 27, 35, 37, 39, 41, 51, 53, 64, 65, 67, 69
speculation, 9
stabilization, 10
stress factors, 52
structuring, 17
successful aging, 39, 57
survival, 11, 25, 37, 40, 43, 47, 58, 59, 68
survivors, 60
susceptibility, vii, 19, 52
syndrome, 32, 64, 73
synthesis, 23, 31
systemic lupus erythematosus, 47

T

T cell, 14, 18, 27, 31, 60, 63, 71, 73
T lymphocytes, 68, 70
T regulatory cells, 63
telomere, 9
temperature, 43
tension, 7
therapy, 45, 70
thyroiditis, 32, 69
tissue, 25, 28, 53, 54
TLR, 14
TLR2, 20
TLR3, 64
TLR4, 20, 24
TNF, 20, 21, 33
training, 52, 53, 76, 77
transcription, 31, 33, 34, 68, 70
transduction, 31, 66
translocation, 31
trauma, 25, 67
tryptophan, 44
tumor, 14, 15, 20, 27, 38, 48, 64
tumor necrosis factor, 20, 48, 64
type 2 diabetes, 47

U

urinary tract, 1

V

vaccine, 47, 63
variations, 18, 43, 45, 68
vein, 68
viral infection, 19, 47
viruses, 13, 59
vitamin C, 50, 51
vitamin E, 50, 51, 75
vulnerability, vii, 1, 15, 19

W

wealth, 52
wear, 10

Y

young adults, 23, 39, 66

Z

zinc, 51